15A

Acc. No. 712/cat

Der 10599   T
£15-95

10 0337687 6

Understanding Pain and its Relief in Labour

KT-149-303

DATE DUE FOR RETURN

RARY

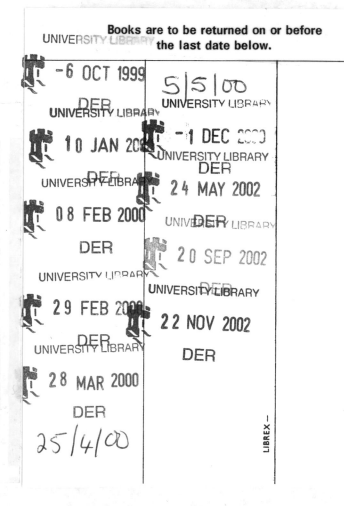

To my mother, Caroline and Paul

For Churchill Livingstone

Editorial director (Nursing and Allied Health): Mary Law
Project manager: Valerie Burgess
Project development editor: Dinah Thom
Design direction: Judith Wright
Project controller: Derek Robertson
Page layout: Kate Walshaw
Copy editor: Adam Campbell
Indexer: Janine Fearon
Promotion executive: Hilary Brown

Understanding Pain and its Relief in Labour

Edited by

Sue Moore MSc BA RGN RM
Senior Lecturer, School of Women's Health,
University of Central England in Birmingham,
Birmingham, UK

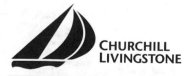
CHURCHILL
LIVINGSTONE

NEW YORK EDINBURGH LONDON MADRID MELBOURNE SAN FRANCISCO AND TOKYO 1997

CHURCHILL LIVINGSTONE
Medical Division of Pearson Professional Limited

Distributed in the United States of America by
Churchill Livingstone, 650 Avenue of the Americas,
New York, N.Y. 10011, and by associated companies,
branches and representatives throughout the world.

First published 1997

ISBN 0 443 05026 0

British Library Cataloguing in Publication Data
A catalogue record for this book is available from
the British Library.

Library of Congress Cataloging in Publication Data
A catalog record for this book is available from
the Library of Congress.

Medical knowledge is constantly changing. As new
information becomes available, changes in treatment,
procedures, equipment and the use of drugs become
necessary. The editors, contributors and publishers
have, as far as it is possible, taken care to ensure that
the information given in this text is accurate and up
to date. However, readers are strongly advised to
confirm that information, especially with regard to
drug usage, complies with the latest legislation and
standards of practice.

The
publisher's
policy is to use
**paper manufactured
from sustainable forests**

Produced through Longman Malaysia, PP

Contents

Contributors

Fiona Alderdice BSSc PhD
Research fellow,
Health and Health Care Research Unit,
The Queens University of Belfast, Belfast UK

Thelma Bamfield BA(Hons)
Senior Lecturer (Midwifery),
University of Central England in Birmingham,
West Midlands, UK

Ruth Bevis RGN RM RHV ADM
Formerly Anaesthetic Sister (Midwifery)
at St Michael's Hospital, Bristol, UK

Lesley Choucri BSc(Hons) RM RGN ADM
FETC(730)
Practice Development Midwife,
Calderdale Healthcare NHS Trust,
Halifax, West Yorkshire, UK

Rosalind Davies MCSP SRP IFA
Senior Obstetrics and Gynaecology
Physiotherapist, Birmingham Women's Hospital
NHS Healthcare Trust, Birmingham, UK

Linda Hayes MA(SocSci)
Senior Lecturer in Women's Health,
University of Central England in Birmingham,
West Midlands, UK

Miranda Holden ADPA(Aus)
DipNaturopathy(Aus) DMSC(USA)
Private Practitioner, Oxford, UK

Sally Marchant RGM RM ADM
Dip(Research Methods)
Research Midwife, National Perinatal
Epidemiology Unit, Oxford, UK

Sue Moore MSc BA RGN RM
Senior Lecturer, School of Women's Health,
University of Central England in Birmingham,
West Midlands, UK

Preface

Support and care in labour is only one aspect of the childbearing continuum; nevertheless it is a highly significant element of each woman's overall pregnancy and birth experience. Memories of labour and the moment of birth, the events and people surrounding it, remain with a woman for the rest of her life, whether the overall experience is perceived as positive or negative.

As a newly qualified midwife, I learnt that pain in labour could best be relieved by the administration of Entonox or pethidine. As I gained experience and confidence, particularly when supporting women who had their babies at home, I began to trust a woman's ability to give birth without intervention, and often without the need for any pharmacological pain control. The experience of seeing a baby arrive following a drug-free labour and gaze into its mother's eyes, appearing both calm and alert, is truly marvellous. Seeing the mother's joy and satisfaction with such an experience is in turn a privilege for me. Midwives' skills, including those of empowerment and advocacy, can, of course, enable women to achieve a similar experience in a hospital environment.

Naturally, not every woman will benefit either physically or emotionally from a drug-free labour. Labour is one of the most severe forms of pain, and the majority of women will need some assistance. An important aspect of midwifery care is to help the labouring woman obtain the right method of pain relief at the right time.

My continuing professional education and practical experience, especially during my years as a community midwife when I was working with women on a one-to-one basis, led me to question and explore many areas of practice, but none more so than the control of pain in labour. I have also come to recognise that women's needs in labour are often not clearly identified, and even when they are recognised they are not always addressed. Midwives are now working towards giving women continuity of care, control and choice though childbearing (Department of Health 1993), a philosophy which is central to my beliefs about midwifery and, therefore, to this book.

There are many unanswered questions relating to our understanding of pain associated with labour. Since becoming a midwife teacher I have developed a special interest in this area, especially in the psychological aspects of pain in labour on which I based research undertaken for a Master's degree. This book has been inspired by that interest and has largely come into being as a response to students who often lament the lack of texts specifically written for midwives on the subject of pain in labour. Although there are researchers who have examined some areas of labour pain, there is still a dearth of literature dealing with women's experiences. Midwives have tended to focus attention on the pharmacological methods of pain control. With the rising interest in complementary methods of pain management in labour, there appears to be little written on the exploration and evaluation of the effectiveness of these as well as the more traditional methods of pain control. This book is therefore seen as a means of raising some of the issues which need further research as well as a resource for current information relating to the physiology, psychosocial issues and control of pain in labour.

The aim of this book is, consequently, to provide some knowledge and understanding of pain and its application to labour. The significance of the midwife's role in supporting a woman throughout this physiologically and emotionally demanding time is emphasised. In addition, the current methods of pain control are identified. It is anticipated that midwives will be encouraged to continue researching the many factors which influence pain and pain perception in labour, as it must be remembered that this book will not provide all the answers but will hopefully initiate the questions.

Finally, I would like to acknowledge and give thanks to all the women and their families who have provided me with the rewards of being involved in their care during their pregnancies and the births of their children, my friends and colleagues over the years with whom discussion and the sharing of knowledge have helped to raise questions in my mind, and also the students who have been inquiring and challenging, and have thus motivated me to look for the answers.

Birmingham 1997   S.M

REFERENCE

Department of Health 1993 Changing childbirth, Part 1. Report of the expert maternity group. HMSO, London

1

Introduction

Sue Moore

LEARNING OUTCOMES

At the end of this chapter the reader will have

- **an introduction to the themes within the book**

- **an increased awareness of some of the psychosocial factors which influence pain perception**

- **an increased awareness of the approaches adopted in relieving pain in labour**

- **considered the themes from *Changing Childbirth* (DoH 1993) relating to pain relief and care in labour.**

During childbirth, a woman is perhaps more vulnerable than at any other time in her life. The care and support she receives during the birthing experience, and the accompanying emotional outcome, may impinge on her attitude towards her immediate mothering role, and can potentially have more long-term adverse effects (Brazelton 1973, Paykel et al 1980). The midwife is the professional who provides support for the majority of women during pregnancy, labour and the postnatal period, advising and informing throughout. She is also the main person in attendance at more than 75% of births in the UK. *Changing Childbirth* (Department of Health 1993), the report of the Expert Maternity group, is now policy for the provision of all maternity services, and by definition sets an agenda for change. Midwifery, therefore, is currently going through one of its most challenging periods, as proposals which support the implementation of 'woman-centred' care are introduced throughout the UK. The requirement to identify and meet the needs of women who use the maternity services has never been so great. In light of these current challenges, the need for a midwife who possesses the skills that enable her 'to accept responsibility for professional development and to apply knowledge and skill in meeting the needs of individual groups throughout antenatal, intranatal and postnatal periods' becomes apparent (UKCC 1994).

Giving birth is one of the most significant events in any woman's life. It is the transition from womanhood to motherhood, the initiation into 'family' life, the miracle of creating life itself. Birth is the beginning of a partnership between mother and newborn. Every midwife will be aware of the pleasure, excitement and anticipation that a woman brings with her as she enters pregnancy. There are, however, also feelings of anxiety, sometimes unhappiness, sadness and even fear. In fact, it is in sharing these emotions and experiences that the midwife genuinely becomes 'with woman'. It is the midwife who will support and advise the woman in preparation for her role as a mother. The midwife is the professional who will support her throughout labour, whatever the outcome. The majority of women can expect a healthy infant to arrive at the end of an uncomplicated labour. Even for that small proportion of women who need some form of medical intervention in their labour, or assistance with the delivery of the infant, the midwife is invariably the provider of care. She is the person who will be at the woman's side throughout her labour, whatever the environment, whether it is in hospital or at home, and whether or not she has the support of a partner, her family or a friend.

PAIN IN LABOUR

Care during the intrapartum period has traditionally been the focal point of midwifery practice. This is a time of extreme need for women in labour, both physically and psychologically. The time surrounding birth engenders conflicting feelings of excitement, apprehension, uncertainty and joy. The woman approaching birth is eagerly awaiting the arrival of her baby, she is wanting labour to be a positive experience, and yet she is uncertain about how she will cope with the pain. She knows that she will survive, being aware that women do not die from the pain of childbirth, and knowing that many forms of pain relief are available if she needs them.

The management of pain during labour usually involves the use of pharmacological methods of pain relief. The routine use of such methods has arguably been brought about by the belief that labour pain is, like pain experienced in many clinical conditions, both unwanted and unnecessary. Melzack & Wall (1988) suggest that 'despite the obvious progress in our knowledge, many people who suffer cancer pain, post-operative pain, labour pain and various chronic pains are inadequately treated' and that 'every human being has the right to freedom from pain'. There can be no doubt that there is a need to improve the quality of life of individuals suffering from cancer pain or chronic pain; however, whether labour pain should be perceived in the same way as these other conditions is debatable. Current trends in the demand for 'natural' childbirth and the use of water immersion during labour suggest that there are many women who feel it appropriate to experience labour without pharmacological pain relief.

It has been shown that a totally pain-free labour, as facilitated by epidural anaesthesia, is not necessarily synonymous with a satisfying event (Morgan et al 1982). Morgan et al's study demonstrated that epidurals are extremely effective in producing a pain-free labour, but that during the early postnatal period some women felt that they had 'had the birth taken away from them' and were left with 'no sense of achievement', leading to dissatisfaction with the experience. Since Morgan et al's study, there has been very little research which explores further the relationship between pain relief and satisfaction with the experience. The ability to recognise the needs of the woman during pregnancy, and throughout the process of birth, and to anticipate her adjustment to motherhood in the postnatal period are accepted parts of the midwife's role. It is also acknowledged that these needs are many and varied.

The following chapters will address, in the main, one specific area of need: the preparation for, and relief of, pain in labour. The knowledge and skills that the midwife requires to support a woman at this time are diverse and include the following: aspects of physiological, sociological and psychological processes; a development of appropriate interpersonal skills and attitudes in communicating with the woman and her family; an understanding of the need for practice based on sound research evidence; an empathic understanding of the labour process; and a knowledge and understanding of all the methods available to relieve the woman's distress should the pain surpass her ability to cope.

Pain in labour is unique, in that it is normal and not the result of some pathological condition. Although it is essential that midwives are able to detect any deviation from normal progress in labour, pain is not a symptom used to diagnose illness. However, it is helpful to explore some of the issues relating to pain associated with ill-health in order to increase understanding of the debates which exist around pain management during labour. To this end, Chapter 2 introduces some of the debates surrounding the various explanations for pain and pain perception.

TOWARDS AN UNDERSTANDING OF PAIN

There have been attempts to understand and explain pain throughout history. The work of famous 19th century scientists such as Muller and Von Frey led to a greater understanding of physiological processes. However, the limitations of many of these scientific theories are apparent when the complex issues surrounding the subjective experience of pain and the differing needs of individuals in treating pain are considered. It became increasingly apparent that pain could not be explained by a simple process of stimulation of specific nerve pathways. It wasn't until the middle of the 20th century that researchers began to propose theories which acknowledged and might explain some of the complex phenomena associated with pain perception.

Midwives are now regularly meeting an informed, questioning client group and are therefore required to have an in-depth knowledge and understanding of the labour process. Every midwife must be able to recognise the 'common factors which contribute to, and those which adversely affect, the physical, emotional and social well-being of the mother and baby' (UKCC 1993). In labour this can only begin with a knowledge and understanding of the physiological processes involved. Chapter 3 presents an introduction to the physiology of pain transmission, and covers the application of this knowledge to labour. Studies on the physiological processes associated with pain in labour are at present relatively few in number, the majority of work having been undertaken by physiologists using animal models. It is assumed that the reader has at least a basic knowledge of the main anatomical structures within the central and peripheral nervous system.

PSYCHOSOCIAL ASPECTS OF PAIN IN LABOUR

The study of the psychology of pregnancy and childbirth has provided many explanations for individual responses to pain as well as the factors which influence the way women cope with labour pain; some of these are presented in Chapter 4. Psychology may be described as the scientific study of both experience and behaviour. Studies in psychology attempt to explain how people think, how individuals develop their particular attitudes or beliefs, what makes people behave in the way they do, and what influences that behaviour. Melzack (1984) suggests that pain associated with childbirth is one of the most intense forms of pain, and this is demonstrated in Figure 1.1 which compares pain scores relating to many serious conditions, such as arthritis, cancer and fractured limbs.

Psychological methods of pain relief are often regarded as secondary to the traditional pharmacological methods. However, there are those who now question the safety of analgesic and anaesthetic drugs (Wagner 1993). In fact, the World Health Organization issued a policy statement that the routine use of 'analgesics and anaesthetic

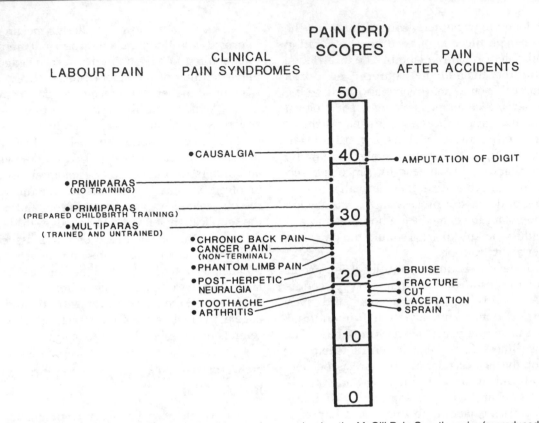

Figure 1.1 Comparison of pain scores (including labour pain scores) using the McGill Pain Questionnaire (reproduced with kind permission from Wall & Melzack 1994).

drugs which are not specifically required to correct or prevent complications at delivery should be avoided'. The side-effects of the more commonly used drugs on both mother and infant are well documented. Most drugs cross the placental barrier, and the short- and long-term effects on the baby have at times been debated. The growing belief in the effectiveness of non-pharmacological pain relief has highlighted the importance of appreciating the psychological processes involved.

The sociological context has over the years had a great influence on the provision of pain relief in labour. There exists a disparity between the culture of traditional midwifery practice and the modernist culture of scientific traditions which brought about the concept of 'medicalised' childbirth. Many have challenged the practices which were implemented as a result of this 'medicalisation', particularly the various interventions in

labour. Medicalisation of maternity care has therefore been identified by some feminist authors as evidence of a patriarchal system, with its inherent drive for power and control (Oakley 1984, Garcia et al 1990). Throughout this century an increasing dependence on the pharmacological management of pain has become apparent. Chapter 5 is a sociological perspective of the factors that have influenced the rise of various methods of pain relief since the mid-20th century. This chapter is based on a current study of women's experiences of labour and birth by Thelma Bamfield, and illustrates the development of some of the ideologies surrounding the management of childbirth in modern times. For a long time, the provision of effective medical care was considered by many to be the only element of importance in the care of women during pregnancy and parturition. Much current evidence, however, suggests that there are other significant factors, such as social and economic influences, which have an effect on the well-being of mothers and their infants. Environmental factors are therefore now included in the criteria for reducing maternal and perinatal morbidity and mortality rates, and not just the intensification of medical intervention (Townsend 1985).

There is currently a growing recognition of the particular needs of women from certain ethnic minority groups using the maternity services (Combes & Schonveld 1992, Department of Health 1993). Antenatal and postnatal care are now considered to be areas in which more effective organisation and management will help in meeting such needs. Furthermore, the needs of these women during labour is an area which has, as yet, not been well addressed. In Chapter 6, Linda Hayes introduces some of the issues identified in the literature which influence the type of care received by Asian women in labour. Some local initiatives have begun to identify ways of improving access to effective care—for example, through the use of link-workers and interpreters—however, such initiatives are in their infancy. Access to support workers for these women during labour is even more limited because it would require a 24-hour service.

It is also recognised that there are many other cultures who have 'special needs' for which there is very little research available. Ethnic groups vary in their customs, preferences, beliefs, values and moral codes, leading to cultural variation in the subjective experience of pain perception and pain behaviour. Problems are frequently encountered when ethnocentric views by other groups or individuals lead to prejudice and discriminatory behaviour. For example, it is not an uncommon belief that women of certain ethnic groups experience pain in labour differently from others, and that specific vocalisations are 'part of their culture'. Such views, particularly if held by midwives or other professionals caring for women in labour, may potentially lead to a belief that these women do not need the same level of pain relief as others, as it is 'expected of their culture'. This could be prejudicial and very misleading; each individual's sensory experience is unique. It is how they behave and cope with the pain that is

more readily influenced by culture. As such, professional attitudes towards certain groups of women could result in them not receiving appropriate pain relief during labour.

THE MIDWIFE'S ROLE

Midwives need to be aware of current research and to increase their knowledge as developments in understanding occur. As the main providers of care in labour, midwives are also in a position to examine the processes associated with labour and the physiological factors which influence the subjectivity of pain perception. It is often through observing how women respond to pain in labour, by listening to the woman's own experience and by identifying the effects of various forms of pain relief, that knowledge of pain processes is increased.

Chapter 7 introduces an analysis of midwifery care through a study conducted by Lesley Choucri. The themes of this chapter relate to aspects of control and empowerment of women as seen from their own and a midwife's perspective. The interactions between midwives and the labouring women which 'enable' or 'disable' the women's feelings of control over events and their experience of pain are presented. This chapter is not directly about pain, but it is about the factors which influence pain perception and labour experience. In presenting the findings of her research, Lesley provides an opportunity for midwives to reflect on some of the issues relating to the skills of being 'with woman'.

NON-PHARMACOLOGICAL RELIEF OF PAIN IN LABOUR

Traditionally midwives provided holistic care for women in labour, acknowledging not only their physical needs, but also their emotional and spiritual needs. Women are once again seeking the forms of care that address such needs. 'Midwives were the great priestesses of the ancient worlds, encouraging women during their first major challenge: the birth ceremony. Through massage, herbs, prayer, and sweat baths they prepared women to embrace the goddesses accompanying the sun from its celestial height to its setting low over the earth' (Stapleton 1995). Complementary therapies are growing in popularity, as women reclaim control over their own childbearing experience and midwives regain the skills of being with woman.

Chapter 8 draws on some of the knowledge presently available surrounding the use of complementary methods of pain relief in labour. Aromatherapy, reflexology and acupuncture are methods of reducing pain in labour which have become accessible to women as midwives have trained and gained experience in their use. Many other methods are currently available through practitioners of complementary medicine, some of whom take a particular interest in providing care for women throughout childbearing. However, the majority of complementary medicine is only available outside the NHS. This in itself may limit access for many groups of women. Midwives and therapists are currently striving to work together to 'integrate complementary therapies into the National Health Service' (Mason 1995).

An area associated with the relief of pain in labour which has been particularly in focus in recent years is the use of water, or hydrotherapy. In April 1995, an international conference on water-birth brought together some very eminent proponents of the use of water for labour and birth from all over the world. Birth in water was, after all, a natural consequence for women who were using water pools as a method of pain relief in labour. Literature surrounding the use of water in labour is growing and so too is the provision of water-birth facilities for women in labour. Although the debate about birth in water continues, there are many who have faith in the effectiveness of hydrotherapy for pain relief.

Midwives are rising to the challenge of implementing *Changing Childbirth* (Department of Health 1993), and midwifery-led maternity units are increasingly providing woman-centred care. Many such units have been striving to ensure that women experience childbirth positively, and in the process are introducing a more conducive environment including the installation of birthing pools. The work of the National Perinatal Epidemiology Unit (NPEU) has been effective

in collating and coordinating much of the available evidence throughout England and Wales (Alderdice et al 1995). Chapter 9 draws on the findings of this survey and will help any midwife currently needing appropriate information for identifying possible advantages and disadvantages of the use of water in labour. It also identifies the main areas of the literature to be consulted when setting up further research into the practice of labouring and giving birth in water. Midwives wishing to provide women with the soothing, pain-relieving effect traditionally associated with the use of water in labour will find this chapter particularly helpful.

Transcutaneous electrical nerve stimulation (TENS) is a method of pain relief which is gradually becoming available to women in many labour environments. The knowledge acquired from one area of practice where the use and effectiveness of TENS in labour has been researched is presented in Chapter 10. Ros Davies, in her role as an obstetric physiotherapist, has worked consistently to provide training for midwives in the use of TENS, as well as educating women themselves about the use of TENS in labour. Ros therefore presents some helpful information for anyone setting up a training programme, or who may want to increase their knowledge of TENS.

PHARMACOLOGICAL METHODS OF PAIN RELIEF IN LABOUR

The majority of women in labour will nevertheless use one of the pharmacological methods of pain relief. The National Birthday Trust Study reported that 60% of women used Entonox for pain relief in labour, 37% used pethidine and 18% used an epidural (Steer 1993). The frequency of use of other methods of pain relief, as identified by the women and their midwives in this particular survey, is shown in Table 1.1. These results also illustrate midwive's apparent disregard of relaxation as a method of pain relief in labour. A midwife, as a practitioner of normal midwifery and someone who is trained to administer analgesic medicine, must be 'fully instructed in its use and familiar with dosage and methods of administration or application' (UKCC 1993).

Table 1.1 The frequency of analgesic methods recorded by the women, their midwives or both (reproduced with kind permission from Chamberlain et al 1993)

Method	Women		Midwives		Both	
	n	(%)	n	(%)	n	(%)
Entonox	3665	(60.0)	5706	(55.1)	2700	(74.0)
Pethidine	2247	(36.9)	3918	(37.8)	1783	(79.4)
Relaxation	2073	(34.0)	406	(3.9)	143	(6.9)
Epidural	1178	(19.3)	1834	(17.7)	872	(74.0)
Massage	1178	(19.3)	515	(5.0)	174	(14.7)
TENS	335	(5.5)	428	(4.1)	235	(70.0)
GA	238	(3.9)	82	(0.79)	17	(7.1)
Diamorphine	128	(2.1)	375	(3.6)	83	(65.0)
Meptazinol	107	(1.8)	337	(3.3)	80	(75.0)
Homeopathy	22	(0.4)	21	(0.2)	5	(23.0)
Hypnosis	4	(0.07)	1	(0.01)	1	(25.0)
Acupuncture	1	(0.02)	2	(0.02)	1	(50.0)
Total	6093		10 352		6093	

Ruth Bevis identifies some of the most frequently used drugs in Chapter 11, along with their routes of administration, and the most frequently reported effects and possible side-effects.

Regional anaesthesia, including epidural and spinal block, is the single most effective method of total pain relief in labour. There are a proportion of women for whom regional anaesthesia will provide analgesia superior to any other form of pain relief (Morgan 1993). The different types of anaesthesia are identified in Chapter 12. Midwives will continue to support and care for women with an epidural or spinal block in progress. A knowledge of the techniques used by the anaesthetist, as well as any possible complications of regional anaesthesia, is therefore essential. A distinct advantage of regional anaesthesia is its use with delivery by Caesarean section, allowing the woman to be conscious during the operation and thus able to share in the unique moment of the birth of her baby.

CHANGING CHILDBIRTH

The overriding aims of the maternity service must be to provide the pregnant woman and her family with as safe an outcome as possible for her and her baby, to offer her choice in the type of support and care she needs and to ensure she retains control and responsibility. Good maternity care will be built on trust between professionals and women and between the professionals themselves

(Department of Health 1993).

The ethos behind *Changing Childbirth* provides women with the best opportunity for gaining control of their childbearing experience. Midwives are also provided with the facilities for regaining traditional skills and autonomy in supporting the woman. The themes surrounding *Changing Childbirth* are choice, continuity, control and change. These themes are key issues in the development of the knowledge and skills necessary for supporting and advising a woman about pain relief in labour. *Changing Childbirth* is therefore fundamental to this book. By identifying some of the issues surrounding pain perception and the relief of pain, it is anticipated that future midwives will gain the knowledge to become effective carers for women and their families, thereby providing them with a birth experience that will leave them fulfilled and in optimum health, both physically and emotionally.

REFERENCES

Alderdice F A, Renfrew M J, Marchant S, Ashurst H, Hughes P, Berridge G, Garcia J 1995 Labour and birth in water in England and Wales. British Medical Journal 310 (6983): 837
Brazelton T B 1973 Effect of maternal expectations on early infant behaviour. Early Child Development and Care 2: 259–273
Carter L 1994 Taking over. Nursing Times 90 (12): 39–41
Chamberlain G, Wraight A, Steer P (eds) 1993 Pain in its relief in childbirth: the results of a national survey conducted by the National Birthday Trust. Churchill Livingstone, Edinburgh

Combes G, Schonveld A 1992 Life will never be the same again: learning to be a first time parent. Health Education Authority, London

Department of Health 1993 Changing childbirth: report of the Expert Maternity group. HMSO, London

Garcia J, Kilpatrick R, Richards M (eds) 1990 The politics of maternity care: services for childbearing women in twentieth-century Britain. Clarendon Press, Oxford

Mason M 1995 A fertile partnership; the role of aromatherapy in midwifery. Aromatherapy Quarterly 47: 27–29

Melzack R 1984 The myth of painless childbirth. Pain 19: 331–337

Melzack R, Wall P 1988 The challenge of pain. Penguin Books, London

Morgan M 1993 Obstetrical anaesthesia. In: Chamberlain G, Wraight A, Steer P (eds) Pain and its relief in childbirth: the results of a national survey conducted by the National Birthday Trust. Churchill Livingstone, Edinburgh, pp 69–77

Morgan B, Bulpit CJ, Clifton P, Lewis PJ 1982 Effectiveness of pain relief in labour: survey of 1000 mothers. British Medical Journal 282 (11): 689–690

Oakley A 1986 The captured womb: a history of the medical care of pregnant women. Blackwell, Oxford

Paykel E S, Emms E M, Fletcher J, Rassaby E S 1980 Life events and social support in puerperal depression. British Journal of Psychology 136: 339–346

Stapleton H 1995 Women as midwives and herbalists. In: Tiran D, Mack S (eds) Complementary therapies for pregnancy and childbirth. Bailliere Tindall, London, pp 153–180

Steer P 1993 The methods of pain relief used. In: Chamberlain G, Wraight A, Steer P (eds) Pain and its relief in childbirth: the results of a national survey conducted by the National Birthday Trust. Churchill Livingstone, Edinburgh, pp 46–67

Townsend P 1985 Inequalities in health. Penguin Books, London

Wagner M 1993 The birth machine. Temple University Press, Philadelphia

Wall P, Melzack R 1994 Textbook of pain. Churchill Livingstone, Edinburgh

UKCC 1994 The Midwife's code of practice. UKCC, London

UKCC 1993 Midwives' roles. UKCC, London

2

Defining pain

Sue Moore

LEARNING OUTCOMES

At the end of this chapter the reader will have

- **considered the complexities encountered when attempting to define and explain pain**

- **an increased awareness of issues relating to the perception of pain and perception of pain in labour**

- **considered the purpose of pain**

- **an introduction to some phenomena associated with pain and pain in labour**

- **an introduction to the language and measurement of pain**

- **considered some methods of studying pain.**

Any attempt to appreciate the meaning of pain immediately highlights the complexities of the many aspects involved in the transmission, perception and associated experience of pain. Almost every person feels pain, with the exception of the relatively few who are born without the ability to feel any painful sensation, i.e. those with congenital analgesia. Pain, although perceived as unpleasant, is therefore recognised as being essential to life. Those unfortunate individuals suffering from congenital analgesia often die relatively young from the consequences of their disease, for instance from chronic recurrent infections, osteomyelitis or conditions which are left undiagnosed, e.g. a perforated appendix. However, the variation in individual pain experience, together with the fact that every person's perception and ability to cope with pain is different, suggests that pain is not readily explained as a basic physiological process transmitted by specific components within the nervous system. It is interesting that the single word 'pain' is used to describe such a complexity of human experience. Pain, therefore, is a very broad term for a multiplicity of physiological, psychological and sociological events.

This chapter introduces some of the debates and issues identified in the literature relating to pain, as well as a few of the more general concepts associated with pain including some explanations and theories of pain, the purpose of pain, the measurement and study of pain and pain phenomena. Some of these issues are also discussed in the context of pain in labour. Currently, there is a dearth of literature relating specifically to the perception and experience of pain in labour. The need for research and discourse increases as women seek to regain control over the natural processes of childbirth, while at the same time wanting to retain the security so often associated with technological advances and medical intervention.

In the mid-1980s, a subcommittee was appointed by the International Association for the Study of Pain (IASP) in order to define pain so that a common understanding and global definition could be reached. The committee consisted of many eminent people in the field. The definition since adopted and utilised worldwide is as follows:

...pain is an unpleasant sensory and emotional experience associated with actual or potential tissue damage, or described in terms of such damage.

Unlike other definitions the IASP recognised that to limit a definition of pain to a 'sensory experience evoked by tissue damage' (Mountcastle 1980), or 'a pattern of stimuli and responses' (Sternbach 1968) somewhat underestimates the subjective experience, as well as the fact that pain can occur without apparent injury or damage to the body.

PAIN: EMOTIONAL OR PHYSICAL?

Morris (1991) describes 'the myth of two pains' which separates physical pain from mental pain.

Morris proposes that this myth is a 'cultural assumption' which 'blinds us to what we can't explain'. A question is therefore raised as to whether the 'pain' experienced by the death of a much loved child, for example, is 'far more than an empty metaphor'. Emotional pain can be perceived to 'hurt' as much as physical pain. A definition of pain must therefore acknowledge physiological and emotional components.

And yet, a distinction is usually drawn between emotional and physical pain, again illustrating the sort of value judgements that are often made in relation to individual experience. Latham (1988) suggests that 'pain experienced by the loss of a loved one can increase emotional pain felt by a patient but he communicates this as an increase in his physical pain'. Such behaviour suggests that the individual's pain experience will be more readily recognised and acknowledged if he expresses it as physical pain.

PERCEPTION OF PAIN

Pain is a sensory experience and as such is often compared with other sensations such as taste, touch, smell, hearing and vision. However, within the visual system, light stimulates specific receptor cells in the eye which then transmit information to visual centres in the midbrain and on to the visual cortex. Pain is not transmitted by specific receptor cells which are sensitive to pain alone. Pain receptors are widely spread throughout the superficial layers of the skin and are sensitive to different types of stimuli such as mechanical damage, extremes of temperature and chemical substances. The physiological processes are explained in more detail in Chapter 3.

'Perception' generally refers to visual processes; however, it is routinely applied to other sensory experiences, such as pain. Perception is defined as 'the combined processes of selection, organisation and interpretation of sensory data ... it is also influenced by learning, by mental sets and by prior experience' (Koenigsberg 1989). The perception of pain therefore encompasses the subjective component, i.e. the psychological component—the way a person 'sees' pain.

Pain as perceived by others

The assessment of pain as perceived by others has often presented professionals with difficulties as they struggle to alleviate clinical pain conditions, postoperative pain and of course labour pain. It has, for example, been demonstrated that health professionals were not always effective in assessing and treating pain, especially postoperative pain (Royal College of Surgeons and College of Anaesthetists 1990). Similarly, it has been suggested that doctors and midwives caring for women throughout labour may not be adequately assessing true pain experience (Rajan 1993). As Rajan points out, 'professionals were significantly more likely to agree with one another about the effectiveness of pain relieving methods than to agree with the women and were less likely to have responded where the women judged their pain relief poor'. There is therefore a suggestion that assessment of individual pain experience is not always accurate, and is further influenced by the subjectivity of the carer. Subjectivity is the internalisation of beliefs and values held by each person, not always arising from rational thought or objective evidence. Some people will consequently believe that all pain is always unpleasant and should be relieved by whatever means is available. Alternatively, as Balaskas (1989) suggests, pain may be described by women in labour as a 'positive or life-giving' experience, identifying that some women actually feel pleasure as a result of labour pain.

Perceptions of pain in labour

Pain in labour is unique in that it is often perceived as an acceptable or necessary pain. A small-scale study exploring the psychological factors associated with pain in labour examined women's feelings about pain (Moore 1995, unpubl. data). The women in this study all appeared to have realistic expectations of what pain in labour was going to be like, and yet they demonstrated a capacity to perceive labour pain as different from other kinds of pain, supporting the view that labour pain cannot readily be compared with the pain experienced in most clinical conditions. Subjects were asked if they saw labour pain as different from other kinds of pain:

'I think of labour pain as a wonderful thing and having a meaning … What a woman is prepared to go through and usually repeats to have her children is a powerful statement of nature' (subject 13)

'Worth the discomfort, not pain associated with illness but a "natural" event' (subject 4)

'Different because you gain something special at the end of labour' (subject 5)

'Because it's what I call the "unknown", you don't know how, where, when it's going to happen, and mostly all your plans are forgotten … you do depend on other people more than pain relief' (subject 14)

The majority of these women were knowledgeable about pharmacological methods of pain relief in labour. The guarantee of a pain-free labour was not enough to prevent the majority of this subject group from resisting any desire to have an epidural during labour. There are some women, therefore, who have a positive attitude towards labour pain. Midwives and doctors, on the other hand, will be aware of possible negative outcomes of pain experience, and in a caring role will endeavour to protect people from potential adverse psychological consequences. This patriarchal approach is being increasingly resisted as proponents of natural childbirth and pressure groups assert their belief in the normality of uncomplicated childbirth. Pain in normal labour is not associated with physical ill-health; likewise there is no evidence to suggest it is associated with an adverse psychological outcome unless the labouring woman's expectations are not met or are unrealistic.

Such debates can only add to the complexity of pain perception. They may also suggest that labour pain requires a separate definition. However, it is important that midwives acknowledge the individuality of women in labour and that their needs for relief of pain are addressed holistically, recognising the many factors that influence pain perception.

Labour pain signals the onset of established labour. This provides a clue as to why it is acceptable to most women. It is predictable—she knows that it is going to happen and approximately when it will happen. Labour can therefore be self-diagnosed. The woman herself knows what is likely to happen; she can anticipate events, learn about what will happen and identify potential ways of dealing with the pain. The potential 'fear of the unknown', as experienced with many acute clinical conditions, is likely to be less profound for that reason, arguably reducing the distress the woman experiences as a result of labour pain well below what she would feel if, for example, the pain were due to a potentially life-threatening condition. Labour pain is not normally life-threatening; on the contrary, it is life-giving.

PURPOSE OF PAIN

One of the first questions people will commonly ask when thinking about pain is: 'Why do we need it?' In evolutionary terms pain is considered to be advantageous. It initiates a response which enables the individual to immediately withdraw from harm. A child, for example, who touches a hot object that burns, or is pricked or cut by a sharp instrument, will withdraw very quickly and in the process will learn not to repeat the event. Pain and its responses are therefore necessary for survival. Ongoing pain associated with trauma also forces the individual to rest the injured area thus allowing healing to take place. It is perhaps protracted pain which raises most questions about the long-term value of pain. The way in which individuals perceive chronic pain often depends on whether the underlying condition causing the pain is benign or malignant, and whether it is continuous or episodic (Sarafino 1990).

It is chronic pain in particular that medical science struggles to alleviate. Chronic pain is experienced over the long term, it is physically and emotionally debilitating and often difficult to treat. It causes intense suffering in the individual which may progressively worsen. Physiologically, receptors do not adapt to pain sensation as do many other sensory receptors. In fact, in some chronic conditions the pain thresholds become lower so that pain receptors are more easily activated, producing an increased response to painful stimuli, sometimes described as hyperalgesia. In addition, chronic pain is often associated with more severe forms of illness such as

cancer, which in particular prompted Melzack & Wall (1988) to state that they were 'appalled by the needless pain that plagues so many people'. Many would accept that it is these types of pain, which affect every element of life (physical, emotional and social) in an adverse manner, which would seem to have no purpose. Chronic pain is debilitating; it often results in individuals having to give up regular employment, and it may well have a negative influence on social and family relationships as the person becomes increasingly demoralised, and as such can ultimately be seen as both unwanted and unnecessary. Chronic pain is now usually managed in specialist pain clinics which adopt an holistic view of individual circumstances.

Pain in labour

Pain associated with labour and the pattern of pain in labour appear to have a very specific purpose, which can also be understood in evolutionary terms. Labour itself is the active process of delivering a baby which, in the human species, is totally dependent on its mother for survival. Even today, women want to get themselves to a place that they perceive to be safe when they are about to give birth. In early labour, they will usually contact the people who are going to support them throughout the birthing process. They then have an opportunity to prepare themselves emotionally, as well as physically, for the birth of a helpless infant who will need protection from harm. It is arguable, therefore, that women who wish to come into hospital in early labour are responding to a basic instinctual drive. For others a safe environment will be their home, surrounded by people they know. To be discouraged from seeking their own perceived 'safe environment' may inevitably increase emotional distress, thus heightening pain perception, even in early labour.

PHENOMENA OF LABOUR
Precipitate labour

Considering the physiological processes that are involved in labour, it is hard to imagine that it could be painless. Yet most midwives will have cared for a woman who has experienced a precipitate labour. Although relatively rare, there are some women who are completely devoid of any labour sensation, and are only aware of imminent birth because of an inevitable awareness of the second stage, as the baby begins to emerge. These women are often shocked and at risk of obstetric complications such as postpartum haemorrhage, as they had little opportunity to adapt to the physiological and psychological processes of labour. They look back on the event frequently, and remember it in very negative terms. In these cases, the infant is often also extremely shocked due to the rapid delivery. It would seem, then, that pain-free labour is not desirable. It has also been suggested that the increased perception of unpleasantness in these cases is associated with the body's inability to release endorphins, the body's 'natural opiates', which normally create a sense of well-being in addition to relieving pain (Robertson 1994).

Fetus ejection reflex

Odent (1987) has described this 'contradictory phenomenon' in which an adrenaline response, instead of inhibiting labour as may be expected, precipitates delivery of the infant. Midwives will be aware of situations in which certain threats to a labouring woman can bring about delivery. Women have sometimes responded to the threat of a forceps delivery, for example, with what appears to be a 'last effort' which results in them rapidly giving birth. Newton (1987) suggests that the term 'fetus ejection reflex' itself emphasises the importance of the psychological aspects of a mechanism that has traditionally been studied as a physiological phenomenon. In studies on animals, Newton demonstrated how animal mothers were able to regulate labour so that the young were born in a safe, quiet environment. The mother inhibited birth in the first stage of labour if placed in threatening conditions, and yet, if constantly disturbed, labour was dramatically speeded up, resulting in delivery of the young after an initial delay. This demonstrates the relevance of environmental factors on labour.

Although these experiments were conducted on animals, most midwives will recognise similarities with patterns of labour in women. It is not unusual for a woman's labour to stop when she comes into hospital, nor is it unusual for a woman quickly to reach the second stage of labour if the midwife, in whom she has built trust and rapport, is soon to be going off duty. The fetus ejection reflex is often preceded by a period of extreme agitation and apparent loss of control. As Odent says, the woman will often use 'frightening words to do with death or suddenly behaves as if she is angry'. This can, of course, be very distressing not only for the woman but also for her birth supporters and carers, as she appears to be in excessive pain. Labour normally follows a pattern in which pain, associated with contractions, acts as an indicator of progress, providing some degree of reassurance that in most cases labour is progressing steadily and safely. The possible consequences of adverse environmental influences are also evident. It is important that the labouring woman is disturbed as little as possible and is free from constant interruptions, particularly from staff in the labour ward or unplanned visitors and birth attendants.

EXPLAINING PAIN

Over the years, there have been varied attempts to explain pain perception.

Specificity theory

The idea of a single pain pathway transmitting noxious stimuli to centres in the brain was the basis of some of the original explanations of pain transmission and perception. 'Specificity theory' suggests that pain is a specific sensation arising as a result of injury, and that sensory information is carried through the peripheral and central nervous systems via pain receptors in the periphery and specific pain nerves in the spinal cord. Specific pain pathways then transmit pain information via specific nerves in the thalamus to specific regions in the cerebral cortex where pain is finally analysed. The problem with this explanation is that it does not take account of the different types of pain experience and the individuality of pain perception, nor of the fact that pain pathways do not transmit pain in isolation.

Pattern theory

Whereas specificity theory proposed that a specific pain sensation system exists within the body, 'pattern theory' suggests that no separate sensory system for pain exists and that pain receptors and pathways are shared with other sensory experiences such as touch. Pain normally arises from injury, resulting in what is referred to as organic pain. There are, however, occasions when an individual feels pain without any apparent reason. This type of pain is usually referred to as psychogenic pain, i.e. it is psychological in origin. There are many who would say that such pain is not 'real'; however, this raises once again the question of whether emotional pain should be regarded as being less profound than physical pain, or whether psychogenic pain should be relieved using the same methods of treatment as are used for organic pain.

Gate-control theory

Many theories may at first hand appear to be adequate explanations of pain transmission and perception. Physiologically, pain transmission is conveyed along neural pathways within the nervous system. However, it is worth considering some of the treatments used to relieve certain chronic pain conditions, which have been founded on beliefs that specific pain pathways transmit pain. Surgical techniques which divide the nerve pathways that transmit pain have often proved ineffective as the pain frequently returns or appears in another area. Such remedies have often been based on a reductionist view that places greater significance on physiological explanations for all bodily functions. It is now more commonly recognised that explanations for pain perception must be addressed from both physical and psychological perspectives.

Melzack & Wall introduced the 'gate-control theory' as an explanation for pain perception in 1965. This theory now provides a comprehensive explanation for both physiological pain transmission and the psychological components of pain, as well as explaining the modulation of pain. The gate-control theory helps to explain the effectiveness of various methods of pain relief, such as massage and transcutaneous electrical nerve stimulation (TENS), as well as the 'placebo' effect. Melzack and Wall have modified the theory since it was first proposed. Although it does not yet explain completely every aspect of pain, it is currently the most readily accepted explanation. The physiology of the gate-control mechanism is explained in more detail in Chapter 3, and its application in the use of TENS is explained in Chapter 10.

TYPES OF PAIN

Pain sensation is diverse. Pain felt when a person breaks an arm or leg is very different from pain due to a burn; similarly, pain experienced in labour is usually perceived as very different from pain associated with toothache. Midwives are often asked by pregnant women what the labour pain is going to be like. Professionals taking antenatal classes have been known to compare labour with other common pains such as toothache or menstrual pain, but such a simplistic view is unrealistic. Women should be presented with an honest notion of what pain may be like, without provoking unnecessary distress. Every woman should be given adequate information so that she can make an informed choice about what methods of pain relief she may want to use. It is not easy for one person to communicate the real meaning of pain to another, nor is it easy to identify a single factor that will predict a woman's experience of pain, but there are certain psychological characteristics which may help (see Ch. 4). It is part of every midwife's role to adequately prepare a woman for childbirth. Midwives can only give adequate information on an individualised basis by getting to know the woman, by understanding her social and cultural background, and by recognising some of those individual characteristics which will help her to explore how she is likely to perceive labour pain, as well as how she may best cope with it.

EFFECT OF PREVIOUS PAIN EXPERIENCE

Niven (1990) points out that pain may be 'exacerbated by acute and illogical anxiety', particularly if that anxiety is created by previous experiences of pain. Niven's study in fact found that women's previous experience of pain, including menstrual pain, is likely to influence their perception of pain in labour in an inverse way. It was shown that women who had experienced severe pain before, including severe dysmenorrhoea, suffered significantly lower levels of labour pain than those who had suffered more moderate pain previously. These findings are contrary to the popular opinion that people who experience high levels of pain on previous occasions will subsequently suffer intense pain. One of the proposed explanations is that women who have experienced severe pain previously have learned how to cope with their high levels of pain using strategies such as relaxation and distraction.

PAIN THRESHOLDS

Variation in pain experience is frequently explained by differences in pain threshold. It is important to distinguish between different pain thresholds, which are measured experimentally and demonstrate physiological changes. Midwives will often refer to a woman's pain 'threshold' when describing her ability, or more often her inability, to tolerate severe levels of pain, i.e. they will say she has either a 'high' or 'low' pain threshold. Four thresholds have been identified by Melzack & Wall (1988) and these are illustrated in Box 2.1. The sensation threshold has been demonstrated to be similar in most individuals. Variation in pain perception is therefore related to differences in the other thresholds. Pain perception thresholds and pain tolerance thresholds have been shown to vary among certain cultural groups. In the context of labour, the encouraged pain tolerance threshold is the level to which women can be encouraged to tolerate labour pain by, for example, reassuring support and effective antenatal preparation. A woman who is aware that she may be able to tolerate a

---

Box 2.1 Pain thresholds (after Melzack & Wall 1988)

Sensation threshold:
the lowest value at which stimulation is felt, e.g. a tingling or warmth

Pain Perception threshold:
the value at which stimulation feels painful

Pain Tolerance threshold:
the level at which the subject wishes to withdraw from the stimulation

Encouraged Pain Tolerance threshold:
the level to which the subject can be encouraged to tolerate stimulation, i.e. to higher levels than the pain tolerance level

---

higher level of pain than she anticipates before labour will gain confidence in her ability to cope, thus enabling her to feel more in control of events.

PAIN RELIEF OR PAIN EXACERBATION?

The experience and perception of pain in labour can add to the complexities so far identified. Labour pain, unlike most other pain conditions, can be considered to be normal—it is not pathological in origin, i.e. it does not result directly from injury or disease. There is, however, the potential for trauma as a consequence of labour, particularly as a result of certain interventions, such as episiotomy and instrumental delivery, or as a result of perineal lacerations sustained during the second stage of labour. The experience and the consequences of such pain cannot be underestimated, particularly in the postnatal period. MacArthur et al (1990) have demonstrated long-term morbidity in many women following epidural anaesthesia. Dewan et al (1993) have also shown that postpartum pain, in the form of uterine cramps, perineal pain and breast pain, presented potential difficulties for women on their return to normal activity following the birth. They also demonstrated evidence to support MacArthur's findings concerning long-term backache following epidural anaesthesia. The need for every midwife to be aware of the potential long-term consequences of forms of care and intervention in labour is apparent, particularly as such consequences can paradoxically result from certain methods of pain relief.

LANGUAGE OF PAIN

The English language can be quite limited when it comes to conveying the meaning of pain. As described previously, the single word 'pain' encompasses a vast amount of complex human experience. However, there are some common descriptors of pain which are used frequently: 'I have a throbbing headache'; 'I called the doctor because I had this stabbing pain in my stomach'; 'my toothache felt as though it was gnawing away in my head'. Pain in labour also has associated characteristic, sometimes emotive, words and phrases (Table 2.1): 'the pain was very strong, but it came in short bursts'; 'it started as a low cramping, ache, then gradually got stronger'; 'it was gruelling, I thought I was dying'. Such language aids the assessment of the type and intensity of the pain sensation.

Melzack & Torgerson (1971), in the initial stages of a study, asked subjects to categorise 102 of the most commonly used words into small groups. The results from this study demonstrated three major dimensions associated with pain: sensory, affective (emotional–motivational) and evaluative. These three classifications relate to the following (Melzack & Wall 1988):

Table 2.1 Descriptions characteristic of clinical pain syndromes[1] (including menstrual pain and labour; reproduced with kind permission from Wall & Melzack 1994)

Menstrual pain (n =25)	Arthritic pain (n =16)	Labour pain (n =11)	Disc disease pain (n =10)	Toothache (n =10)	Cancer pain (n =8)	Phantom limb pain (n =8)	Postherpetic pain (n =6)
Sensory							
Cramping (44%)	Gnawing (38%)	Pounding (37%)	Throbbing (40%)	Throbbing (50%)	Shooting (50%)	Throbbing (38%)	Sharp (84%)
Aching (44%)	Aching (50%)	Shooting (46%)	Shooting (50%)	Boring (40%)	Sharp (50%)	Stabbing (50%)	Pulling (67%)
		Stabbing (37%)	Stabbing (40%)	Sharp (50%)	Gnawing (50%)	Sharp (38%)	Aching (50%)
		Sharp (64%)	Sharp (60%)		Burning (50%)	Cramping (50%)	Tender (83%)
		Cramping (82%)	Cramping (40%)		Heavy (50%)	Burning (50%)	
		Aching (46%)	Aching (40%)			Aching (38%)	
			Heavy (40%)				
			Tender (50%)				
Affective							
Tiring (44%)	Exhausting (50%)	Tiring (37%)	Tiring (46%)	Sickening (40%)	Exhausting (50%)	Tiring (50%)	Exhausting (50%)
Sickening (56%)		Exhausting (46%)	Exhausting (40%)			Exhausting (38%)	
		Fearful (36%)				Cruel (38%)	
Evaluative							
	Annoying (38%)	Intense (46%)	Unbearable (40%)	Annoying (50%)	Unbearable (50%)		
Temporal							
Constant (56%)	Constant (44%)	Rhythmic (91%)	Constant (80%)	Constant (60%)	Constant (100%)	Constant (88%)	Constant (50%)
	Rhythmic (56%)		Rhythmic (70%)	Rhythmic (40%)	Rhythmic (88%)	Rhythmic (63%)	Rhythmic (50%)

[1] Only those words chosen by more than one-third of the patients are listed and the percentages of patients who chose each word are shown below the word.

1. Words that describe the sensory qualities of the experience in terms of temporal, spatial, pressure, thermal and other properties.
2. Words that describe affective qualities in terms of tension, fear and autonomic properties that are part of the pain experience.
3. Evaluative words that describe the subjective overall intensity of the total pain experience.

In the second part of this study, certain subclasses were identified, and these included words such as 'hot', 'burning', 'scalding' and 'searing'. The majority of subjects were in agreement about the order in which these words described intensity of pain.

MEASUREMENT OF PAIN

It was the realisation that many people use the same words to describe pain that eventually led to the development of the McGill–Melzack Pain Questionnaire (Fig. 2.1). Melzack was then a professor at McGill University in Montreal, Canada— hence the term McGill Pain Questionnaire (MPQ). Each person undertaking an assessment of his or her pain is instructed to select from each section the word that best describes the pain. Each word has an allotted score, depending on the level of intensity of pain described for each section. For example, in the first section, 'pounding' would be scored highest and 'flickering' lowest, and so on. Eventually an overall score, or pain rating index (PRI), is obtained. In addition, the overall pain intensity is assessed by means of the present pain intensity (PPI). This associates levels of pain with a number from 0 to 5: 0 = no pain at all; 1 = mild pain; 2 = discomforting pain; 3 = distressing pain; 4 = horrible pain; and 5 = excruciating pain. Use of the MPQ enables clinicians or researchers to quantify individual pain experience, particularly in terms of pain intensity. The MPQ does, however, have some limitations. It is presumed that English is the main language spoken by the person responding. It also uses some words that may not be readily understood by many English speakers, for example 'lancinating'. The use of these typical pain descriptors has helped doctors in the treatment of chronic pain conditions, as well as facilitating ongoing study into painful conditions.

Another well known method of assessing pain is by the 'visual analogue scale' (VAS). This is a simple technique which requires the person to rate their level of pain intensity on a scale from 'no pain' to 'pain as bad as possible' (Scott & Husskinson 1976). The scale is represented by a horizontal straight line measuring exactly 10 cm. The person marks a point on the line which she believes best represents her level of pain (Fig. 2.2). These scales are easy to use, and have even been used effectively for assessing children's pain.

Both the MPQ and the VAS have been used in research to assess pain in labour (Niven 1990, Melzack et al 1991). However, it is important to recognise the potential limitations of such tools when used in this respect. Pain in labour is not consistent; it gradually changes in nature as contractions of the uterus increase in length, strength and intensity. The MPQ and the VAS best measure pain intensity; it is important therefore to consider at what stage of labour such measures are to be used. The pattern of labour makes it extremely difficult to measure individual pain experience at its most intense, i.e. at the height of a contraction, and towards the end of the first stage of labour.

Measuring pain in labour

Midwives and other professionals require methods for accurately assessing a woman's level of pain. The difficulty in assessing pain arises not so much in identifying whether it is present or not, but in determining how bad it is (i.e. the intensity of the pain) and therefore what type of analgesia will best treat it. In the first instance, it would seem to be most apt to assess a woman's pain by simply asking her how bad the pain is, or whether she is in need of pain relief. Observing labour for typical patterns of 'behaviour' will help the midwife to assess progress in labour as well as the woman's ability to cope with pain. Pain behaviour is described in more detail in Chapter 4.

Communicating with the labouring woman is therefore a fairly obvious method of assessing pain. Nevertheless, it must be remembered that

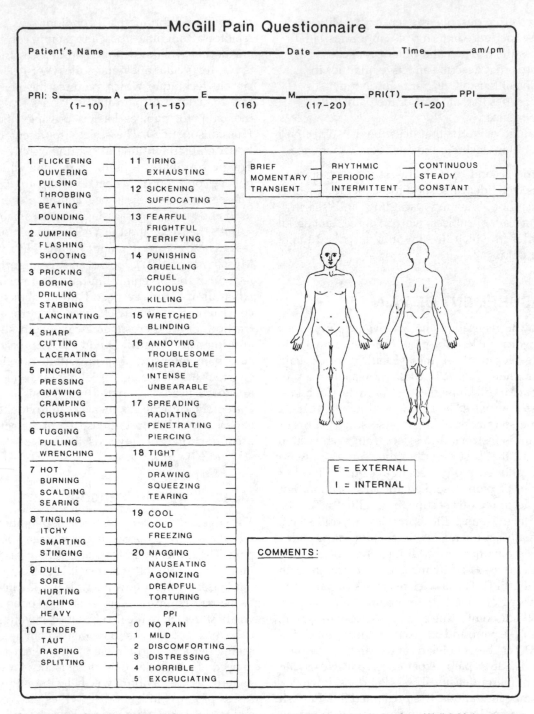

Figure 2.1   McGill–Melzack Pain Questionnaire (reproduced with kind permission from Wall & Melzack 1994).

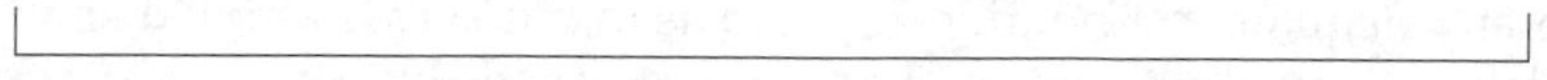

No pain

Pain as bad
as possible

Figure 2.2 Visual analogue scale.

knowing a person is in pain is not the same as assessing the degree of pain. As discussed previously, some studies have demonstrated that professionals are not always in agreement with the individuals actually experiencing the pain. As a result, women may receive inappropriate or ineffective pain relief.

The findings of the National Birthday Trust (NBT) survey (Chamberlain et al 1993) suggest that aspects relating to accurate assessment of pain in labour need further consideration. Poor communication was the most common reason cited by women for their dissatisfaction with the professionals' assessment of their pain. Another common cause of dissatisfaction with the labour experience was the non-administration of an epidural that had previously been promised, and one of the main reasons for this was the unavailability of an anaesthetist. The next national survey to be undertaken by the NBT will be within 10 years. There is a distinct need for further examination of women's experiences of pain in labour before this next survey.

PAIN 'PHENOMENA'

There are certain well-known aspects of pain perception and experience which are difficult to explain. These anomalies are illustrated by those clinical aspects of pain sometimes referred to as the phenomena of pain. Phantom limb pain, for example, is a syndrome in which an amputee continues to feel the presence of an amputated limb; a proportion of these people perceive extreme pain in the non-existent limb. Common sense would suggest that there is no obvious explanation for this phenomenon as there is no clear source of pain. This pain often proves difficult to relieve.

Another example of a pain phenomenon is that of referred pain, alternatively described as mislocation of pain. An example of this is pain experienced as a result of angina or during a heart attack when pain from the damaged heart muscle is referred to the left shoulder and down the arm. Following pelvic surgery, many gynaecological patients will complain of referred pain, which is felt in the shoulder and often described as 'shoulder-tip' pain. One explanation for referred pain is that nerve fibres in the autonomic nervous system, which innervate internal organs, converge in the spinal cord with sensory nerve fibres of the body surface. Another explanation is that, embryologically, the organs and skin areas developed from the same tissue (Rutishauser 1994). Thus the brain interprets signals from internal organs, which cannot be readily translated in the cerebral cortex, as if they were arising from body surfaces, which are more easily interpreted. The characteristics of referred pain can be used in clinical situations to aid in diagnosis of conditions such as pelvic disease, angina or appendicitis, especially as the relationship between internal organs and certain dermatomes is well defined (see p. 31).

There are also many examples of situations in which a person's perception of pain, and reaction to it, is not what is expected. Soldiers in battle who are seriously injured and fight on, seemingly feeling no pain, and certain tribal traditions which require demonstrations of bravery such as walking on burning coals, typically illustrate some of these anomalies relating to pain perception. Conversely, there are some individuals who experience a great deal of pain with no apparent injury. The pain experienced by sufferers of trigeminal neuralgia, pain associated with the fifth cranial nerve, is often described as excruciating. Other types of neuralgic pain, such as that following an attack of a viral infection, herpes zoster, can be very severe, often inconsistent with the amount of infection, damage or injury. The existence of these phenomena makes it more difficult to provide an adequate explanation for pain perception. 'Pain research, it appears, has not yet advanced to the stage at which an accurate definition of pain can be formulated. However, the continuing debate on a definition of pain is a sign of the vigour, excitement and rapid development of the field' (Melzack and Wall 1988).

Placebo

The placebo effect has been the subject of much debate. Wall (1992) suggests that attempts to address the subject often provoke 'a shudder of discomfort like a cold hand in the dark'. The term placebo is derived from the Latin meaning 'I will please'. A placebo drug is a chemically inert drug, usually made up of sugar or salt, which is given as a form of medication, particularly for the relief of pain. The reason that this topic provokes so much debate is that placebo drugs are often extremely effective in relieving symptoms. Many explanations for the effectiveness of placebo have been proposed, including the suggestion that people who respond to placebo have nothing wrong with them in the first place, that there is statistically a fixed proportion of the general population who will respond to placebo (i.e. one-third of any population), and finally that there is a common misperception that giving a placebo is the same as doing nothing and therefore some conditions are likely to resolve spontaneously anyway. It must be acknowledged that the placebo response is not the same phenomenon as relief from the condition. Wall challenges these explanations as 'myths which have been generated in an attempt to preserve the logic on which favoured therapy is based'. It would therefore seem that placebo methods of pain relief are in themselves a form of treatment. Placebo is known to be more effective under certain conditions, for example when given by injection.

Intracutaneous injections of sterilised water Some Scandinavian countries use intracutaneous injections of sterilised water as an analgesic during labour. This technique involves the injection of about 0.01 ml of water, applied in two to four places around the lumbosacral and suprapubic regions where labour pain is felt most strongly.

The injections are applied so that a 'white papule becomes visible with a red zone surrounding it' (Trude et al 1990). This creates an intense burning sensation which lasts 15–20 seconds, with the analgesic effect following some 2–3 minutes later (Trude et al 1990, Trolle et al 1991). This effect can be explained by the gate-control theory (see p. 35), but Trude et al also suggest a placebo effect. They propose that intracutaneous injections are 'a legitimate new type of analgesic'. The advantages of intracutaneous injections are that there is little drowsiness and women can move about freely, the baby is not affected, the pain relief commences rapidly and the treatment can be repeated several times. No apparent disadvantages have yet been identified. There have been no reports as yet of this method being used in the UK.

It can be argued that many methods of pain relief involve a placebo effect, including some of the complementary therapies. And yet the credibility of placebo treatments is less than that of traditional pharmacological methods of pain relief. This does not appear to be purely an ethical issue—the placebo effect works only if the recipient believes in it. Morris (1993) points out that: 'medicine does not quite know what to make of placebos. Normally the placebo effect gets dismissed as merely an annoying variable in pharmaceutical research ... yet the placebo attests to the mind's forgotten power over illness.'

THE STUDY OF PAIN

Any research which examines pain, and more specifically the study of pain in labour, must address many of the complexities previously identified. Pain is a subjective experience. The measurement and comparison of individual pain experience in human subjects raises many ethical and technical problems, some of which will have been apparent in the preceding text. Traditionally experimental studies investigating physiological processes associated with pain transmission have been conducted on animals, particularly rats. The 'tail-flick' test is one such experiment, whereby a stimulus such as heat, known to be painful in humans, is applied to the animal's tail. The time taken for the rat to flick its tail to escape the painful sensation is measured. It is therefore the rat's avoidance of the painful stimuli which is being measured. The effectiveness of many pain relieving drugs have traditionally been studied using this type of test.

As with any research which involves the detailed examination of physiological processes, ethical issues are raised. At one time it was assumed that animals could not feel pain, yet it is recognised that they respond to painful stimuli by withdrawing, in the same way as humans. It had even been assumed, until very recently, that premature newborn babies were not capable of feeling pain because of the immaturity of the nervous system. Yet current research has demonstrated that certain behaviour, such as facial expression, is indicative of pain sensation (Martin et al 1995). The development of measures such as the Liverpool Infant Distress Score for postoperative pain in neonates undergoing corrective surgery is also a fairly recent advance (Horgan et al 1995). The belief that if a recipient of noxious stimuli does not verbalise pain then pain is not being felt has led to many ethical debates in the past. The recognition and assessment of pain in neonates have led to very effective management of pain relief for the sick infant.

Studies conducted on adult human volunteers include the measurement of stimulation of nociceptors as a result of pricking the skin, pressure and application of extremes of heat and cold. A technique known as the 'muscle-ischaemia procedure' has also been used to simulate and examine the experience of pain as felt, for example, during a heart attack. In this technique a sphygmomanometer cuff is applied to the arm and inflated to a level at which pain is produced. Pain thresholds can be measured using this technique, as can an individual's response to the pain.

The study of pain in labour frequently involves the use of animal models, including rats, dogs and ewes. Whether the results from studies using animals can be directly related to human experience is, of course, part of continuing debate. Human subjects have been recruited for some studies (see Ch. 3). The value of objective scientific study has always been emphasised in areas

of research, thus perpetuating the need for experimental studies. The study of pain in labour, whether that be the physiology of pain, or the perception or experience of pain, would need to acknowledge all the potentially influencing variables, e.g. variation in physiological structure (individual differences in size), environmental influences, personal characteristics, social and cultural variations, etc. Midwives are in an ideal situation to add to the body of knowledge through both experimental and, perhaps more readily, observational qualitative study of women's experiences of pain in labour, and also to explore the beliefs, particularly relating to approaches of care, as well as the many factors which influence pain relief.

SUMMARY

It is essential that midwives understand the complexities associated with defining and understanding pain. It is only in this way that they will be able to interpret what a labouring woman is trying to communicate and therefore how best to go about trying to help that woman to be as comfortable as possible. In this respect, midwives must also acknowledge that every woman perceives pain differently, so that they can adjust their methods to suit each case.

REFERENCES

Balaskas J 1989 New active birth: a concise guide to natural childbirth. Thorsons, London
Chamberlain G, Wraight A, Steer P 1993 Pain and its relief in childbirth: the results of a national survey conducted by the national birthday trust. Churchill Livingstone, Edinburgh
1989 Churchill's Medical Dictionary. Churchill Livingstone, Edinburgh
Dewan G, Glazener C, Tunstall M 1993 Postnatal pain: a neglected area. British Journal of Midwifery 1(2): 63–66
Horgan M, Choonara I, Glenn S 1995 The development of a scale to measure postoperative pain/distress in the neonate. Society for Reproductive and Infant Psychology, 15th Annual Conference
Latham J 1987 Pain control. Austen Cornish, London
MacArthur C, Lewis M, Knox E G, Crawford E S 1990 Epidural anaesthesia and long-term backache after childbirth. British Medical Journal 301: 9–12

Martin R, Glenn S, Padden T, Berry N 1995 The pain expression and its genesis in premature infants. Society for Reproductive and Infant Psychology, 15th Annual Conference

Melzack R, Torgerson W S 1971 On the language of pain. Anaesthesiology 34: 50–59

Melzack R, Wall P D 1965 Pain mechanisms: a new theory. Science 150: 331–356

Melzack R, Wall P 1988 The challenge of pain. Penguin Books, London

Melzack R, Belanger E, Lacroix R 1991 Labour pain: effect of maternal position on front and back pain. Journal of Pain and Symptom Management 6(8): 476–480

Morris D B 1993 The culture of pain. University of California Press, Berkeley

Mountcastle V B 1980 Medical physiology. Mosby, St Louis

Newton N 1987 The fetus ejection reflex revisited. Birth 14 (2): 106–108

Niven C 1990 Pain in labour. In: Faulkner A, Murphy-Black T (eds) Excellence in Nursing Research the Research Route. Scutari Press, London

Odent M 1987 The fetus ejection reflex. Birth 14(2): 104–105

Rajan L 1993 Perceptions of pain and pain relief in labour: the gulf between experience and observation. Midwifery 9: 136–145

Robertson A 1994 Empowering women: teaching active birth in the 90's. Ace Graphics, Sevenoaks

Royal College of Surgeons and College of Anaesthetists 1990 Commission on the provision of surgical services. Report of the working party on pain after surgery. RCS and RCAnaesth., London

Rutishauser S 1994 Physiology and anatomy: a basis for nursing and health care. Churchill Livingstone, Edinburgh

Sarafino EP 1990 Health psychology: biopsychosocial interactions. John Wiley and Sons, New York

Scott J, Husskinson E C 1976 Graphic representation of pain. Pain 2: 175–184

Sternbach R A 1968 Pain: a psychophysiological analysis. Academic Press, New York

Trude A, Vegard D, Einar L 1990 The International Confederation of Midwives 22nd International Congress

Trolle G B, Moller M, Kronborg H, Thomsen S 1991 The effect of sterile water blocks on low back pain. American Journal of Obstetricians and Gynaecologists 164: 1277–1281

Wall P 1992 The placebo effect: an unpopular topic. Pain 51: 1–3

Wall P, Melzack R 1994 Textbook of pain. Churchill Livingstone, Edinburgh

3

Physiology of pain

Sue Moore

LEARNING OUTCOMES

At the end of this chapter the reader will have

- **reviewed the main components of the nervous system involved in transmission of painful stimuli**

- **identified the basic anatomy and physiology of neurotransmission**

- **an understanding of the speed of neurotransmission in relation to pain sensation**

- **identified the structure and sensory pathways within the spinal cord**

- **an introduction to the modulation of pain and the gate-control theory**

- **considered the physiological responses to injury**

- **an introduction to some of the physiological mechanisms of pain relief**

- **an increased understanding of the physiology of labour pain**

- **considered some physiologically related processes which influence pain in labour.**

As identified in Chapter 2 the concept of pain is complex. To explain the physiology in traditional terms as a pain pathway along which pain signals are transmitted from the periphery of the body to brain centres is arguably to oversimplify the process of pain transmission and perception of pain.

The human nervous system transmits, processes, analyses and stores all human experience, emotion and behaviour as well as monitoring physiological processes. To identify pain pathways in isolation is therefore potentially to overlook the fact that these other functions are continually taking place. The idea that there are neurones which respond to tissue damage alone is misleading. The following chapter will, however, present some basic information on the structures and processes involved in neural transmission and so aid knowledge and understanding of the pain processes involved in labour. This will include an introduction to the major neural pathways involved in the transmission of noxious stimuli, neurophysiological processes, the physiological modulation of pain, and also the action of some of the more common pain-relieving agents. The physiology of labour pain is not yet well understood; however, what is understood on the basis of the current evidence will also be presented in this chapter.

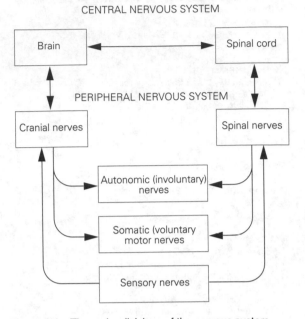

Figure 3.1 The major divisions of the nervous system (reproduced with kind permission from Thibodeau 1992).

COMPONENTS OF THE NERVOUS SYSTEM ASSOCIATED WITH PAIN

The nervous system is made up of two main parts, the somatic and the autonomic nervous systems. The somatic nervous system consists of the sensory, motor and integrative systems, all of which control the relative functions of the body. The somatic nervous system can be further divided into the component parts of the central nervous system and the peripheral nervous system. The central nervous system consists of the spinal cord and the brain. The major structures of the brain are divided into the cerebrum, the cerebellum and the brain stem. The peripheral nervous system comprises all the nerve fibres which are not located in the central nervous system, including sensory nerves, motor nerves, cranial and spinal nerves (Fig. 3.1). The autonomic nervous system comprises the structures that regulate the involuntary functions of the body, such as the cardiovascular system, the endocrine glands, and the respiratory, digestive and urinary systems. Although both somatic and autonomic

nervous systems are involved in the physiology of pain, it is the structures and functions within the central and peripheral nervous systems which will be mainly addressed in this chapter.

Sensory receptors

Sensory information is initially transmitted to the nervous system via receptors in the skin. These receptors are free nerve endings and are widespread in the superficial layers of the skin, as well as in internal structures such as the periosteum (bone tissue), arterial walls and joint surfaces. There are many different types of receptors which are excited by different kinds of stimuli. For example, mechanoreceptors, which are excited by mechanical stress or damage such as pressure or vibration, thermoreceptors which are sensitive to changes in temperature, and chemoreceptors which are sensitive to chemical substances including oxygen, carbon dioxide and water. Chemoreceptors are also sensitive to substances such as histamine, seratonin and bradykinin, which are collectively known as algogens (i.e.

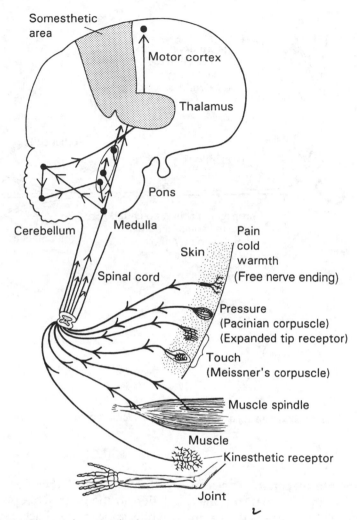

Figure 3.2 Sites at which sensory receptors are stimulated and algogenic substance is released (reproduced with kind permission from Guyton 1987).

'pain producer'). These substances, together with prostaglandins, are released locally within tissue in response to injury (Fig. 3.2). When stimulation such as pressure, heat or cold reaches a certain threshold level, the sensation of pain is transmitted. Sensory nerve endings which respond to noxious stimuli are known as nociceptors; these are free nerve endings situated abundantly throughout the skin, which when activated generate the signals which carry pain information along nerve fibres in the peripheral nervous system to the central nervous system.

Nerve cells and nerve fibres

The basic component of the nervous system and nerve pathways is the nerve cell or neurone (Fig. 3.3). The function of a neurone is to detect the initiation of a sensory signal, to then transmit the information in the form of electrical impulses to other components within the nervous system and so to other systems of the body, such as the musculo-skeletal systems, which then invokes a response. Neurones vary in size and shape depending on where they are situated. Those

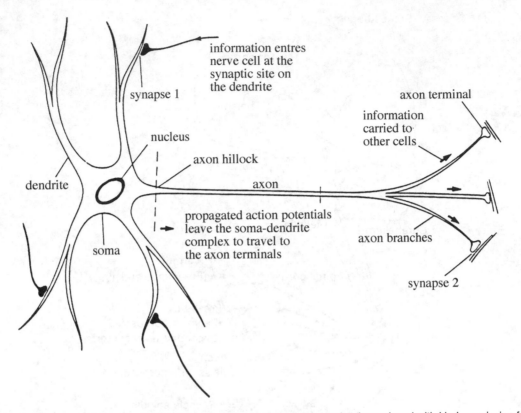

Figure 3.3 The nerve cell (or neurone), illustrating direction of sensory information (reproduced with kind permission from The Open University 1981).

which transmit sensory information from peripheral areas such as the foot to the spinal cord may reach a metre in length. The neurone is typical in that nerve cell processes, termed dendrites and axons, extend from the cell body. The dendrites, forming very fine 'twig-like' structures, pick up information signals, then transmit the signals through the cell body to the axon (see Fig. 3.3). Each axon terminates at the presynaptic or axon terminal. The extracellular fluid which surrounds and bathes all cells has a high concentration of sodium and chlorine, which balances the high concentration of potassium within the cell. This chemical balance is an important function in the transmission of neuronal signals, which is termed neurotransmission.

The axons of nerve cells are surrounded by supporting cells, or Schwann cells. These Schwann cells wrap around a neurone many times, forming the myelin sheath (Fig. 3.4) which acts as an insulation to the axon. This myelin gives the cell a white appearance. Each nerve fibre contains a cluster of axons grouped together as a fascicle. These bundles of nerve fibres are crudely analogous to a typical modern telephone cable, which is surrounded by an insulating coating and contains smaller fibres each of which transmits separate information signals (Fig. 3.5). Nervous tissue which is made up of nerve fibres surrounded by myelin is called 'white matter', and nerve tissue which is made up of unmyelinated axons and cell bodies is called 'grey matter'. The myelin sheath is interrupted at intervals along its length at the 'nodes of Ranvier'. Neuronal impulses, as they are propagated down the axon, jump from one node of Ranvier to the next, i.e. saltatory conduction, which increases the speed of neurotransmission (Fig. 3.6).

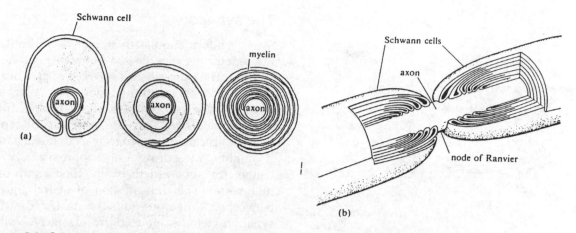

Figure 3.4   Schwann cells forming the myelin sheath around an axon (reproduced with kind permission from The Open University 1981).

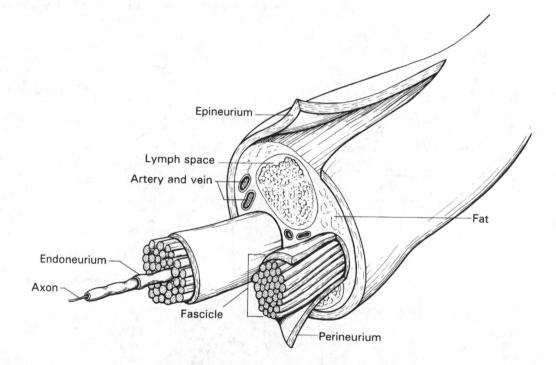

Figure 3.5   A nerve containing axons, which are grouped together as fascicles, which are surrounded by perineurium. Each neurone is surrounded by epineurium (reproduced with kind permission from Thibodeau 1992).

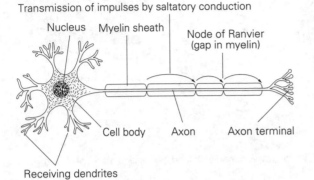

Transmission of impulses by saltatory conduction

Nucleus   Myelin sheath   Node of Ranvier
(gap in myelin)

Cell body   Axon   Axon terminal

Receiving dendrites

Figure 3.6   Neurotransmission: propagation of impulses along an axon (reproduced with kind permission from Voke 1986).

The synapse

Sensory information such as pain is transmitted through the nervous system from one neurone to the next. The transmission between each neurone takes place at junctions known as synapses (Fig. 3.7). The gap between one nerve cell (presynaptic neurone) and the next (postsynaptic neurone) is called the synaptic cleft; the distance is minute, measuring only approximately 20 nanometres (one-fiftieth of one-thousandth of a millimetre). The transmission of neural signals between one neurone and the next, across the synaptic cleft, is effected by chemicals called neurotransmitters. Examples of neurotransmitters include noradrenaline, seratonin, dopamine, gamma aminobutyric acid (GABA), substance P, acetylcholine and enkephalins. These transmitters are contained within small sacs known as

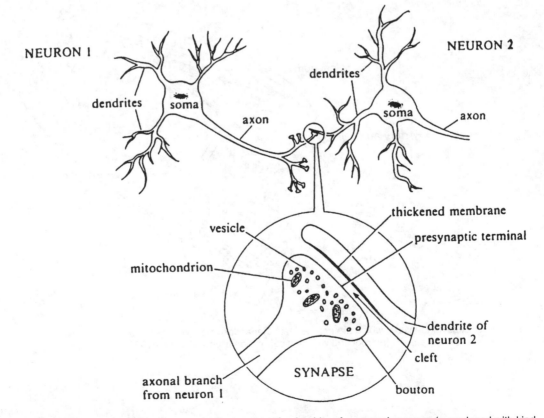

NEURON 1

dendrites   soma

axon

NEURON 2

dendrites

soma

axon

thickened membrane

presynaptic terminal

vesicle

mitochondrion

dendrite of
neuron 2

cleft

axonal branch
from neuron 1

SYNAPSE

bouton

Figure 3.7   A synapse: an axon of one neurone at the junction of a dendrite of a second neurone (reproduced with kind permission from The Open University 1981).

vesicles. When an action potential arrives at the presynaptic axon terminal, the neurotransmitter is released across the presynaptic membrane into the synaptic cleft. The neurotransmitter then diffuses across the cleft to the membrane of the postsynaptic neurone. The postsynaptic membrane contains protein molecules which act as receptor sites at which each neurotransmitter molecule binds (Fig. 3.8). The binding of neurotransmitter molecules and postsynaptic protein molecules stimulates the postsynaptic neurone to initiate conduction of the impulse, transmitting the sensory information, e.g. the pain signal, on its way.

NEUROTRANSMISSION

All cells within the human body have an electrical charge which differs within the cell from the charge outside the cell. Neurones are capable of a 'shift' in charge, moving rapidly from negative (–70 millivolts) to positive (+30 millivolts) and back again, creating an impulse known as an action potential (Fig. 3.9). The action potential is caused by rapid changes in the cell membrane potential. An action potential can be described as a self-propagating wave of electrical disturbance which is transmitted along the surface of the cell membrane. When a nerve cell is 'at rest', the cell is negatively charged. This is known as polarisation. As the cell becomes positively charged, the cell is 'depolarised', allowing the electrical signal, or action potential, to be conducted along its axon. The positive charge on the outside of the neurone's cell membrane is due to an excess of sodium ions (Na^+) on the outer surface of the membrane (Fig. 3.10). When the membrane is stimulated, the permeability is altered so that sodium ions move into the cell. This in turn makes the inside of the cell more positive, the

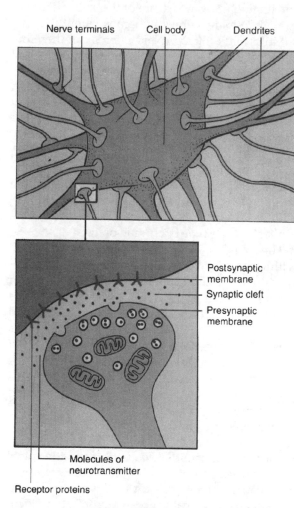

Figure 3.8 Synapses: where they are found and what they consist of (reproduced with kind permission from Rutishauser 1994).

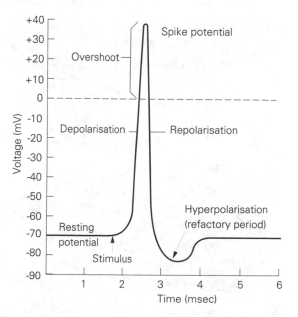

Figure 3.9 An action potential as it is recorded on an oscilloscope (reproduced with kind permission from Voke 1986).

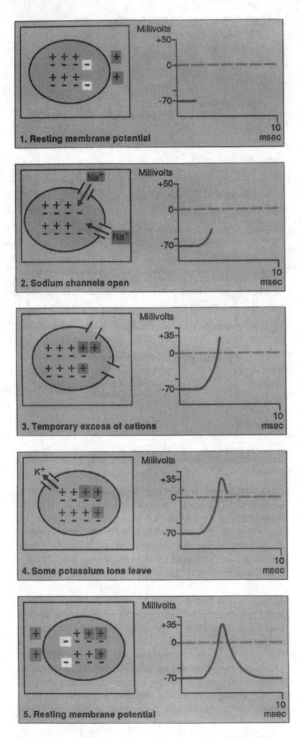

Figure 3.10 The action potential: how the voltage of a nerve cell changes as a result of the opening and closing of sodium and potassium channels (reproduced with kind permission from Rutishauser 1994).

outside then becoming more negative. This change takes place all along the cell membrane, returning to its original state as the impulse passes (Fig. 3.11).

'Fast' (acute) and 'slow' (chronic) pain

In the peripheral nervous system, myelinated nerve fibres are classified as Aβ (A beta) and Aδ (A delta) fibres, whereas unmyelinated fibres are known as C fibres. The larger the diameter of the nerve fibre, the faster is the speed of neurotransmission; however, since myelinated fibres transmit signals faster than unmyelinated fibres, myelinated fibres which are of the same diameter as unmyelinated fibres will consequently transmit information faster. Nerve fibres can therefore be categorised according to their diameter and their speed of conduction (conduction velocity; Table 3.1). It is these two types of nerve fibres, A fibres and C fibres, which give rise to the concept of 'fast' and 'slow' pain. Aδ fibres transmitting 'fast' pain signals at speeds between 4 and 30 m/s give rise to sensations of sharp, well defined, acute pain, which are felt at the time of the actual injury. C fibres transmit 'slow' pain signals at speeds of between 0.4 and 2 m/s and result in pain which is longer lasting, often felt as a 'duller' aching type of chronic pain.

This 'dual' pain sensation is further processed within the spinal cord. The nerve fibres enter the spinal cord and terminate in the grey matter of the dorsal horn of the cord. The Aδ nerve fibres make synaptic connections in the dorsal horn and the brain stem. Signals are then transmitted via nerve pathways such as the spinothalamic tract to the thalamus, from where the information is conveyed to the cerebral cortex (Fig. 3.12). This process of transmission is relatively direct and pain sensation is therefore felt as sharp and well localised. Unmyelinated C fibres also synapse in the grey matter of the spinal cord. Pain sensation is therefore transmitted via C fibres to the spinal cord and then via the spinoreticular tract to the reticular formation and on to the thalamus and cortex. Physiological processes within the reticular formation give rise to stimulation of the nervous system in general, in turn causing symptoms

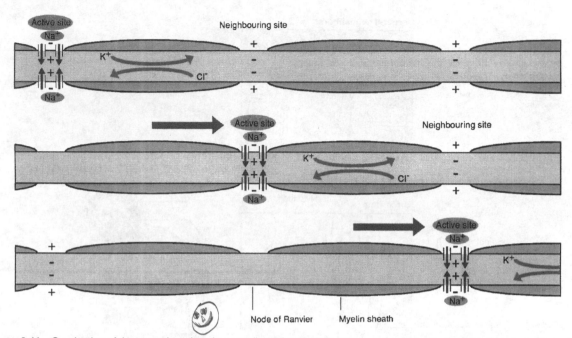

Figure 3.11 Conduction of the nerve impulses in a myelinated axon: how the movement of anions and cations between active and inactive sites depolarises the neighbouring axonal membrane, opens the voltage-gated sodium channels and generates another action potential (reproduced with kind permission from Rutishauser 1994).

Table 3.1 Characterisation of nerve fibres

Type of nerve fibre	Diameter of nerve fibre (μm)	Speed of conduction (m/s)
Myelinated Aβ fibres	5–15	30–100
Myelinated Aδ fibres	1–5	4–30
Unmyelinated C fibres	0.3–1.5	0.4–2

that create a general state of bodily excitement. It is subsequently difficult for the individual to be able to localise this type of very unpleasant pain, and because areas around the basal area of the brain such as the hypothalamus are stimulated, emotional responses are also influenced.

The following sections provide more detail of the distribution of nerves and nerve pathways, demonstrating the route of transmission of nerve impulses between the spinal cord, the brain, and to areas within the body via descending pathways. This will be helpful at a later stage when considering the effect of epidural anaesthesia for pain relief in labour, as well as in understanding the structures involved when the anaesthetist carries out the procedure. Spinal nerves carry

sensory and motor information, therefore influencing not only sensation such as pain, but also movement. Detailed 'maps' of the skin's surface in relation to the source of each spinal nerve and the part of the body which it then innervates are known as dermatomes (Fig. 3.13). An awareness of these sites and the location of the different spinal nerves can help in understanding how doctors can locate spinal cord injury or nerve damage by pricking the related dermatome with a needle to see whether the person is aware of sensation or not. For example, injury or compression to the spinal nerve associated with the first lumbar vertebra, such as is caused by a slipped disc, will cause sensory loss in dermatome L1 (refer to Fig. 3.13).

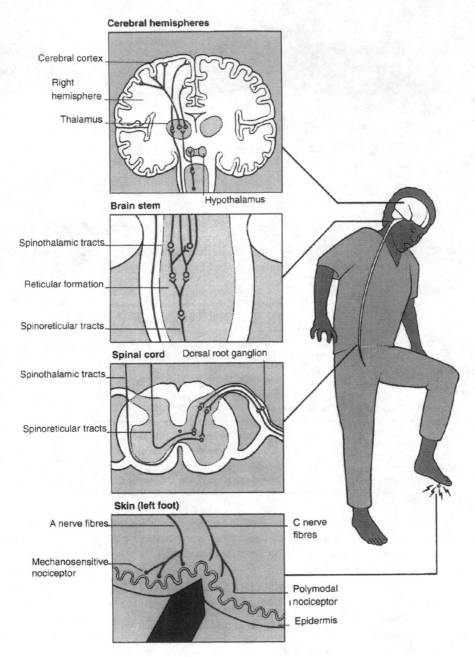

Figure 3.12 Routes through which impulses are transmitted to the brain, giving rise to the sensations of 'fast' and 'slow' pain (reproduced with kind permission from Rutishauser 1994).

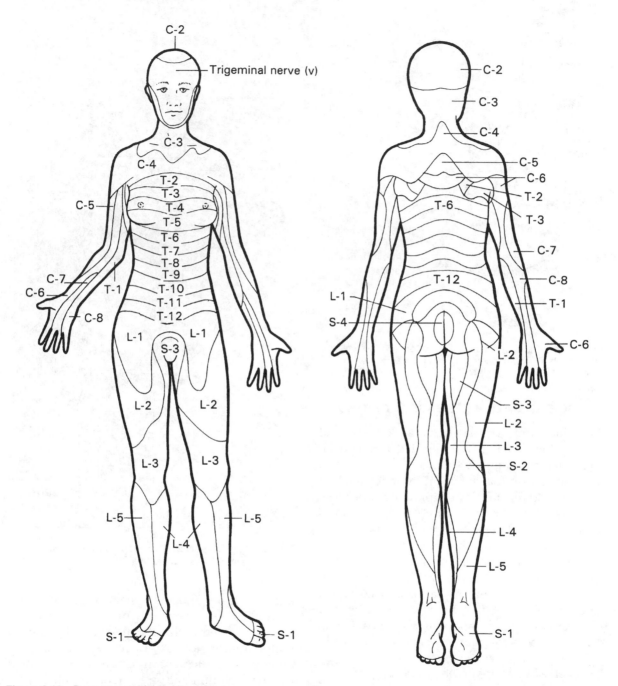

Figure 3.13 Dermatomes of the skin surface.

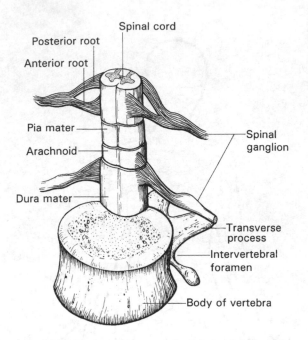

Figure 3.14 The spinal nerves, spinal cord and their relation to the vertebrae (reproduced with kind permission from Thibodeau 1992).

The spinal cord and sensory pathways

The spinal cord is situated within the vertebral column, the spinal nerves leaving through the intervertebral foramina (Fig. 3.14). Once again, this is an aspect that is useful in understanding the siting and functioning of epidural anaesthesia. There are over 30 pairs of spinal nerves, the names of which relate to the level of the vertebral column from which they leave the spinal cord (Fig. 3.15). Therefore, commencing at the neck, cervical nerves arise from cervical vertebrae, and so on through thoracic, lumbar, sacral and coccygeal vertebrae. A knowledge of the location of some of these nerves is very important when positioning TENS electrodes for pain relief in labour.

The internal structure of the spinal cord

The spinal cord is composed of areas of nerve cell bodies (grey matter) and nerve axons (white matter). The cell bodies are arranged centrally in an 'H' shape, which is further subdivided into functional areas called laminae (Fig. 3.16). The function of the grey matter is to relay nerve signals between the peripheral areas of the body

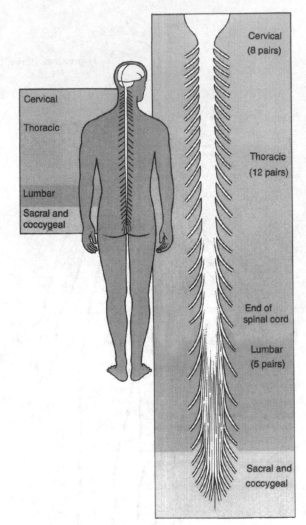

Figure 3.15 The spinal nerves (reproduced with kind permission from Rutishauser 1994).

and the brain, and these signals are relayed in both directions. Sensory information, such as pain, is relayed in the dorsal (or posterior) horn; motor information is relayed in the ventral (or anterior) and lateral horns. There are many small neurones within the grey matter, called interneurones, which transmit signals from sensory neurones to motor neurones. The white matter of the spinal cord is made up of nerve axons which are grouped together into pathways or tracts. These tracts either convey incoming sensory information (afferent) to the brain or carry motor signals away (efferent) from the brain to the

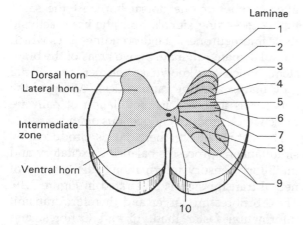

Laminae
1
2
3
4
5
6
7
8
9
10

Dorsal horn
Lateral horn
Intermediate zone
Ventral horn

Figure 3.16 A cross-section of the spinal cord showing regions and laminae, including the substantia gelatinosa. Key: 1. marginal nucleus; 2. substantia gelatinosa; 3 & 4. proper sensory nucleus; 5. zone anterior to 4; 6. zone at base of dorsal zone; 7. intermediate zone; 8. neutral zone; 9. nuclear columns; 10. grey matter surrounding central canal (reproduced with kind permission from The Open University 1981).

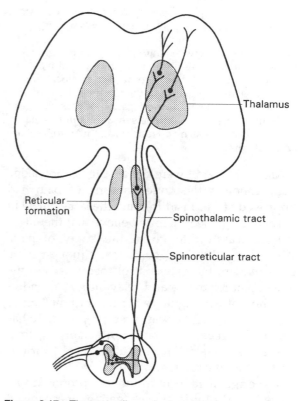

Thalamus
Reticular formation
Spinothalamic tract
Spinoreticular tract

Figure 3.17 The ascending spinal cord tracts.

muscles of the body. The two main ascending sensory tracts are the spinothalamic tract and the spinoreticular tract (Fig. 3.17) which, as identified earlier, are those most usually implicated in the transmission of pain signals.

Pain signals enter the spinal cord via the posterior spinal nerves and are transmitted on into the grey matter of the posterior horn. There are some pain modulating processes which occur at this point before pain signals are transmitted on to the brain. (Much of this processing can be explained by the gate-control theory, which is described in a later section.) Pain signals are then relayed to the brain stem and thalamus. Some of the nerve fibres transmit fast pain to the thalamus along sensory pathways and then signals are transmitted to the sensory cortex, to areas believed to be important for localising pain (Guyton 1987). The fibres which transmit slow pain, on the other hand, terminate mostly in the reticular formation of the brain stem, causing the more general and longer lasting reactions to pain.

Endogenous opioids

Certain neurotransmitters are released at sites within the spinal cord and brain which inhibit rather than activate the conduction of pain signals. These substances are called endogenous opioids. These naturally occurring substances, first discovered in the 1970s, were found in areas of the brain, as well as in the cerebrospinal fluid (CSF) and the blood. Their action is similar to the opiate drugs, such as morphine, as they bind to the same receptors. They are found within neurones and are therefore believed to act in the same way as a neurotransmitter. Many of these endogenous opioids have been discovered, the most important being β-endorphin, enkephalins and dynorphin. It has been suggested that dynorphin is 200 times more powerful than morphine if injected directly into the brain's pain modulating system, and is therefore a very powerful analgesic (Guyton 1987).

MODULATION OF PAIN: THE GATE-CONTROL THEORY

Melzack and Wall first proposed the gate-control theory in 1965. At that time they identified that several facts must be explained by any pain theory, i.e. that (Melzack & Wall 1988):

the relationship between injury and pain is highly variable; innocuous stimuli may produce pain; the location of pain may be different from the location of damage; pain may persist in the absence of injury or after healing; the nature and location of pain changes with time; pain is not a single sensation but has many dimensions; there is no adequate treatment for certain types of pain.

Melzack & Wall were the first to acknowledge that, although the understanding of pain had improved, it was in addressing the last element in particular that led them to believe that there was a long way yet to go in the study of pain. Weisenberg (1994) suggests that although some gaps remain, the gate-control theory is 'still the most comprehensive and relevant for an understanding of the cognitive aspects of pain'. Since the original theory was first proposed, it has gradually developed and now many 'gating' mechanisms are believed to take place at various sites within the brain and spinal cord.

The original gate-control theory proposed that there is a physiological 'gating mechanism' within the substantia gelatinosa of the spinal cord's dorsal horn grey matter. It is suggested that sensory signals can only pass through the cells in the substantia gelatinosa when the 'gate' is open. When the gate is closed, sensory information is blocked, and this forms the basis of a kind of physiological pain relief, i.e. intrinsic to the body.

The opening of the gate is caused by the release of neurotransmitters which excite the postsynaptic membrane of neurones, transmitting pain signals within the ascending 'pain tracts'. The gate is closed by the release of inhibitory neurotransmitters and the release of endogenous opioids (Fig. 3.18). This gating mechanism explains the effectiveness of many pain relieving methods such as rubbing, massage, TENS, as well as many of the psychological methods, e.g. 'mind over matter'.

Activation of the gate mechanism by rubbing, for instance, causes sensory signals to be transmitted by Aβ fibres simultaneously with pain transmission. These Aβ fibres stimulate inhibitory interneurones in the dorsal horn. At the same time, descending signals from the brain activate these interneurones. The descending fibres which modulate pain originate in two areas of the brain stem, which are known as the peri-aquaductal grey matter and the raphe nuclei. Many of the nerve cells involved in modulation of pain are those which produce endogenous opioids.

The gating effect, therefore, is produced by simultaneous processes balancing excitatory and inhibitory sensory information. This balance of neural transmission is illustrated in Figure 3.19. The Aβ fibres are larger and therefore transmit information faster than Aδ and C fibres, and consequently have a dominant effect. These Aβ fibres also release inhibitory neurotransmitters. Rubbing produces stimulation of mechanoreceptors (touch receptors), which activate Aβ fibres causing the gate to close, thus inhibiting pain signals.

THE LIMBIC SYSTEM

The limbic system is an area of the brain which is believed to be implicated in many aspects of human behaviour and experience. It is important to be aware of this area when considering physiological processing of pain together with its emotional effects and consequences, i.e. the psychological aspects of pain. The limbic system is made up of a number of nuclei (groups of nerve cell bodies), and is situated deep in the brain structure. This is an extremely complex system, the function of which is not well understood; however, it has been demonstrated that stimulation of areas of the limbic system in humans can create feelings associated with fear, anger, pleasure and satisfaction. The main structures include the hypothalamus and the amygdala. The hypothalamus is believed to have a relationship with memory of sensory experiences (Rutishauser 1994) and is therefore important in determining learned emotional responses; for example, humans are able to associate pain with previous unpleasant experiences and can therefore learn to avoid these situations in future. The limbic system is therefore believed to be involved in the emotional responses to pain.

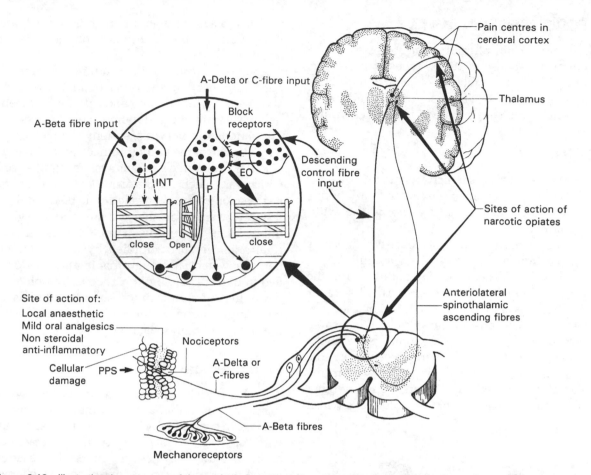

Figure 3.18 Illustrating the gate-control theory: including stimulation of sensory receptors, opening and closing of the pain gate, sites of release of neurotransmitters and endogenous opioids, and ascending and descending pathways. Key: P - substance P; EO - endogenous opiates; INT - inhibitory neurotransmitters; PPS - pain producing substances (reproduced with kind permission from Clancy & McVicar 1992).

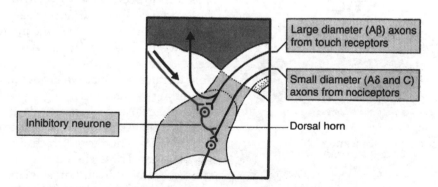

Figure 3.19 Transmission of signals in the pain pathway can be inhibited by simultaneous activity in: (1) other sensory neurones conducting impulses from the skin; and (2) axons conducting impulses from the brain, *both* of which excite inhibitory interneurones (reproduced with kind permission from Rutishauser 1994).

RESPONSE TO INJURY

There are certain physiological processes which occur as a response to certain types of injury. It is useful to have a knowledge of some of these processes in order to increase understanding of responses which are initiated by painful stimuli.

Reflex

There are two reflexes which are initiated by reaction to pain: somatic reflexes and autonomic reflexes. One such somatic reflex is the withdrawal reflex.

A reflex is the automatic response which occurs as a reaction to many types of stimuli, e.g. a painful injury. The neuronal pathway for the most simple type of response is termed a 'reflex arc'. The arc is activated by excitation of a sensory receptor which transmits information via a small interneurone to a motor neurone, causing the muscle to contract and therefore enabling the part of the body affected to withdraw from the cause of injury (Fig. 3.20). There are many other more complex reflexes, for example those which

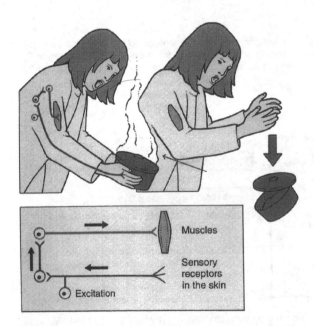

Figure 3.20 An example of a reflex response (reproduced with kind permission from Rutishauser 1994).

maintain balance when a person is pushed, and those which enable the human body to maintain its upright stance.

Autonomic responses (including the 'flight or fight' response), on the other hand, are brought about by sympathetic and parasympathetic reflexes within the autonomic nervous system. The autonomic nervous system is involved in maintenance of the body's homeostasis. In particular, the autonomic nervous system supplies certain organs such as the cardiac muscle of the heart, smooth muscle tissue of the bladder, liver, respiratory and digestive systems, and also glandular tissue. The uterus, a smooth-muscled visceral organ, is also supplied by the autonomic nervous system, although this is seldom identified in most physiology text books. The physiology of the autonomic processes of the uterus will be enlarged upon in the section relating to the physiology of pain in labour.

Physiological

A further initial response to injury is the physiological response that occurs at the time of tissue damage, a process which is particularly apparent with certain forms of injury such as a scratch or an insect sting. For these examples, this reaction is the inflammatory response, and is characterised by redness of the affected area, production of heat, swelling and pain. The inflammatory response is a result of certain physiological processes. Initially, damaged blood vessels go into spasm to prevent blood loss, while at the same time certain substances are released which slow blood clotting; at this stage the injured area often looks white. The area then becomes redder and feels warmer as a result of vasodilation. Serum from leaking capillary walls now causes swelling. Defending white cells (e.g. lymphocytes and macrophages) then begin to destroy cell debris and bacteria. As identified earlier, nociceptors are stimulated by chemicals which are released at the site of injury. These chemicals which include histamine, bradykinin and prostaglandin give rise to sensations which may range from a mild irritation through to a discomfort which is frequently described as pain.

MECHANISMS OF PAIN RELIEF

Three main categories of pain-relieving agents function at certain sites within the 'pathway' of noxious stimuli. Analgesia can first be initiated at the level of the nociceptors by preventing pain sensation from actually occurring and being transmitted along the sensory neurones. Secondly, once an action potential has been initiated along the neural pathway, propagation of the action potential may be blocked, preventing transmission of action potentials. Finally, analgesia may be initiated within the central nervous system. These common modes of pain relief will now be examined briefly in relation to some of the physiological processes which have been introduced in this chapter (see also Chs 11 and 12).

Mild analgesics

As has been described previously, tissue damage causes a certain chemical response at the site of injury. This algogenic response causes the nociceptors in the skin to become activated. Prostaglandins sensitise these nerve endings making them more susceptible to stimulation by the algogenic substances, therefore having a pain producing effect. Mild analgesics such as aspirin and non-steroidal anti-inflammatory drugs (NSAIDs) inhibit the production of prostaglandins, therefore desensitising the nociceptors so that they are less likely to be activated. Paracetamol is also thought to reduce production of prostaglandins, however unlike aspirin it does not reduce prostaglandin production generally, but appears to reduce production in areas of the brain. For this reason paracetamol has less of an anti-inflammatory effect.

Locally acting analgesics (local anaesthetics)

Propagation of action potentials can be prevented by the use of drugs such as lignocaine. Transmission of action potentials involves the movement of sodium ions across a charged cell membrane. Lignocaine blocks the sodium channels of the axon, preventing the action potential from being propagated along the nerve fibre at the site of administration. An injection of lignocaine given to anaesthetise the perineum before performing an episiotomy, for example, will take effect only at the site of injection (unless introduced in error into the general circulation via a blood vessel). Local anaesthetic agents appear to influence C fibres in particular, possibly because they are unmyelinated and therefore more easily penetrated by the drug.

Centrally acting analgesia (narcotics)

The main category of centrally acting pain relieving drugs are the opiates, e.g. morphine and pethidine. These narcotic drugs act on areas of the brain and spinal cord, thus reducing pain perception. Experimental studies using radioactively labelled drugs have demonstrated sites within the central nervous system to which opiates readily bind. These 'opiate binding receptors' have been found in the substantia gelatinosa of the dorsal horn of the spinal cord and also in areas of the brain, particularly the brain stem, and are the sites at which naturally occurring opioids bind. As outlined previously, Aβ, Aδ and C fibres terminate in the dorsal horn of the spinal cord. These fibres then make connections with cells that project to the brain stem conveying sensory information to higher brain centres. Opiates depress the activity of these projecting dorsal horn cells firstly by binding presynaptically to terminals of nerve fibres, thus preventing the release of neurotransmitters which normally produce synaptic transmission. Opiates also increase the activity of descending inhibitory nerve pathways from the brain stem. In addition, opiates act on areas of the limbic system, thereby providing a mood elevating effect.

Other physiological effects of opiates, which any person administering such drugs must be aware of, include depression of the respiratory centres in the medulla, sedation and euphoria, as well as nausea and vomiting (the medulla is also the centre for control of these responses). Opiates may also affect the cardiovascular system. Morphine, for example, may cause bradycardia (slowing of the heart rate). Pethidine, on the other hand, may increase heart rate. Pethidine is the drug most frequently used in the UK for pain relief in labour (see Ch. 11).

LABOUR PAIN: PHYSIOLOGY

Pain in labour has a fairly predictable pattern and is associated with contraction of the uterus. The location of pain sensation throughout labour is continually changing—in duration, degree and frequency—as contraction of the uterus increases. This predictability enables the woman to anticipate and prepare for the arrival of the infant. Initially, pain alerts her to seek a safe place to give birth. Increasing contractions of the uterus with associated pain signal progress throughout the first stage of labour, as descent of the baby and dilatation of the cervix occurs. At the end of the first stage of labour, 'transitional' pain indicates imminent onset of the second stage, the actual birth. It is at this stage that some women find pain extremely difficult to manage and will often ask for pain relief. An understanding of the processes of labour will enable the woman and her carers to cope with this characteristic and overwhelming sensation. Powerful expulsive contractions give rise to a characteristic second stage pain, as the uterus changes its activity to one which enables the woman to actively push the baby into the world. This is an involuntary process and many women are able to negotiate second stage with a minimum of verbal encouragement to 'push' from the midwife. In fact, there is an opinion that this traditional method of instructing the woman to 'take a deep breath, hold it, chin on chest and push' is detrimental to mother and more particularly the fetus, as prolonged breath-holding may cause fetal distress (Caldeyro-Barcia 1979, Sagaday 1995). Furthermore, Bonica (1994) suggests that physical exertion in the second stage as a result of 'active pushing' can cause maternal acidosis. This particular technique for 'managing' the second stage of labour moreover denotes that it is the midwife who is 'in control' of the birthing rather than the woman herself. By encouraging the woman to find her own effective position and to push when her body suggests she should, the midwife will help the woman to be in control of her own labour, a factor which in turn may have an effect on psychologically reducing pain perception and ultimately increasing satisfaction with the experience.

Pain in the first stage of labour

Bonica (1994) provides one of the most comprehensive reviews of the physiological processes involved in labour pain, reporting that the pain in the first stage of labour is due mainly to dilatation of the cervix, as well as to distension and stretching of the lower segment of the uterus. It is also suggested that pain is caused by 'contraction of the uterus under isometric pressure, that is, against the obstruction presented by the cervix and perineum, which is the "adequate stimulus" for provoking pain in hollow viscera'. The uterus is a visceral organ and, as such, Melzack & Wall (1988) suggest that it gives rise to pain only if it is dilated or in strong contraction. Other suggestions include ischaemic changes of the myometrium and cervix, pressure on the sensory nociceptors of the body of the uterus, and also inflammatory changes in the muscles of the uterus (Polden & Mantle 1992).

Bonica (1994) reports a longitudinal study carried out on 305 women in childbirth. Using a discreet local anaesthetic block of nociceptive pathways during labour, he demonstrated that spinal nerves T10, T11, T12 and L1 supply the uterus, including the lower segment, and the cervix. These findings contradict some obstetric and anatomy texts which have in the past identified that the cervix was supplied by sacral nerves.

The peripheral neural pathways supplying the uterus, cervix and perineal structures are shown in Figure 3.21. Aδ and C fibres supplying the uterus and cervix accompany sympathetic nerves which supply the uterus in a particular sequence. Nociceptive nerve fibres from the uterus and cervix pass to the spinal cord through the uterine and cervical nerve plexuses (a network of nerves), the pelvic plexus, the middle and then the superior hypogastric plexuses. These nociceptive nerve fibres then pass through the posterior roots

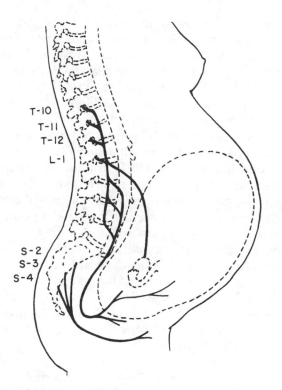

Figure 3.21 Neural pathways supplying the uterus, cervix and perineal structures (reproduced with kind permission from Wall & Melzack 1994).

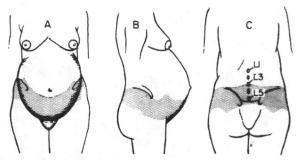

EARLY FIRST STAGE : Pain intensity Moderate

Figure 3.22 Pain intensity and distribution in relation to dermatomes in early labour (reproduced with kind permission from Wall & Melzack 1994).

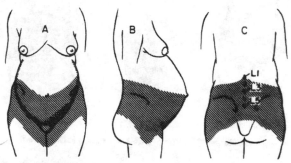

LATE FIRST STAGE : Pain Intensity Severe

Figure 3.23 Pain intensity and distribution in relation to dermatomes in late labour (reproduced with kind permission from Wall & Melzack 1994).

of spinal nerves T10, T11, T12 and L1, to synapse at the interneurons in the posterior horn of the spinal cord. Nerve fibres also travel from perineal structures through the pudendal nerve to the spinal cord through spinal root nerves S2, S3 and S4. The lower lumbar and upper sacral segments also supply pelvic structures which are involved in the pain of childbirth.

As with other types of pain, labour pain is felt over dermatomes supplied by spinal cord segments that receive their stimulation from the uterus and cervix. Pain throughout the first stage of labour is 'referred' to those dermatomes which are supplied by the same spinal cord segments receiving the painful stimuli. In the early first stage of labour, moderate pain is felt in the T11 and T 12 dermatomes (Fig. 3.22). In established labour, more severe pain is felt in the T11 and T12 dermatomes, and it spreads to the T10 and L1 dermatomes (Fig. 3.23).

Pain in the second and third stages of labour

Pain in the second and third stages of labour is different from the first stage. The cervix is now fully dilated and neural stimulation from the cervix decreases; however, contraction of the body of the uterus is maintained. As the presenting part of the fetus descends through the pelvis, pressure on nociceptors throughout the pelvic floor and perineum increases pain in those areas. Pain is further influenced during the second stage by stretching of the pelvic peritoneum and uterine ligaments, stretching of the bladder, urethra and rectum, and pressure on the lumbosacral nerve plexus. An abnormally presenting part, as with a deflexed fetal head in the occipito-posterior position, can increase the pain felt in

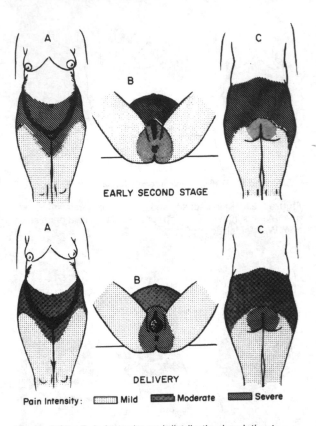

Figure 3.24 Pain intensity and distribution in relation to dermatomes in the second stage of labour (reproduced with kind permission from Wall & Melzack 1994).

these regions throughout the late first stage and second stage of labour. At the end of the first stage and in the second stage of labour, pain is often described as cramping and burning and may be felt in the thighs and legs (Fig. 3.24).

Biochemical changes in labour

Beta-endorphin levels, in particular, are known to increase through labour, and to peak at delivery and during the early postnatal period up to a possible level that is 10 times that of non-pregnant levels. It is thought that other endogenous opioids may also raise the pain tolerance threshold in labour. Bonica (1994) reports on this phenomenon, which is called pregnancy-induced analgesia or 'hypalgesia', suggesting that pain tolerance thresholds normally rise at the end of pregnancy.

Some studies were undertaken using rats to demonstrate this effect (Gintzler et al 1983). Other studies carried out on human subjects during pregnancy demonstrated similar findings using radiant heat to produce noxious stimuli. The suggestion is that pregnancy-induced hypalgesia results from the activity of dynorphin opioid receptor systems in the spinal cord, and is sufficient potentially to lower the intensity of pain in labour. Varassi et al (1989) conducted a small randomised trial, which demonstrated that an exercise programme in pregnancy increased beta-endorphin levels. As well as the general positive physical effects of fitness, the study group ($n = 16$) demonstrated significantly raised beta-endorphin levels, and during labour significantly higher pain scale ratings were recorded by the control group. The increase in beta-endorphin and dynorphin levels would appear to provide some confirmation that there is an intrinsic form of analgesia during childbirth.

Some studies have shown that acute pain produces increases of 20–40% in catecholamine levels (especially noradrenaline as normally occurs in response to stress), which in turn causes a decrease in uterine blood flow (Bonica 1994). There are many potential detrimental effects of labour on the mother and fetus. As outlined in Figure 3.25, an increased sympathetic response will eventually cause increased peripheral resistance, increased cardiac output, and a subsequent rise in blood pressure and raised oxygen consumption by the labouring woman. Hyperventilation will in turn eventually cause respiratory alkalosis in addition to the increasing adrenaline levels and decrease in uterine blood flow. This increased sympathetic activity would appear to provide physiological reasons for the use of systemic analgesics as proposed by Bonica (1994). These potentially deleterious effects would appear to justify Bonica's belief that regional analgesia by means of epidural anaesthesia is the best method for minimising such effects. Epidural anaesthesia has been shown to reduce the release of catecholamines and other neuro-endocrine substances such as cortisol and ACTH. It has, however, also been shown to reduce the release of beta-endorphins. It must be argued that many

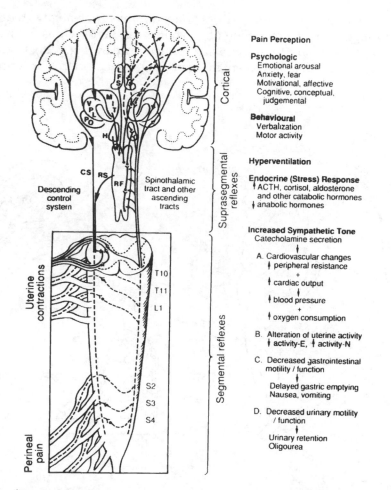

Figure 3.25 Diagrammatic representation of the transmission of painful stimuli to the spinal cord by uterine contractions and perineal pain in the second and third stages of labour. Nociceptive impulses reaching the brain stem provoke cortical responses which include perception of pain, initiation of psychological mechanisms and behavioural responses. RF, reticular formation; RS, reticulospinal; H, hypothalamus; LFS, limbic forebrain structures (reproduced with kind permission from Wall & Melzack 1994).

non-pharmacological methods of pain relief may be potentially as effective in reducing sympathetic responses, particularly as such methods reduce anxiety and stress. A general reduction in anxiety levels, by providing an appropriate environment and support from carers, would therefore appear to be advantageous to mother and fetus. Women can manage pain in labour with no adverse consequences using relaxation techniques together with other non-pharmacological and psychological methods, if that is what the woman believes in and trusts. This is an area that requires more research evidence.

Influence of maternal position in labour

Many of the studies investigating the physiological processes of labour have been conducted on women who have had continuous cardiotocography, as well as eventual systemic analgesia and epidural anaesthesia. It would be of interest to consider the position these women are bound to adopt throughout their labour, as it can reasonably be assumed that they would be fairly restricted in their movement. As indicated previously, the maternal position in labour might have a great influence on a woman's experience of pain. Simkins (1989) suggests that a reduction of painful stimuli can be achieved by, for example, changing the maternal position and movement in labour, thus potentially reducing mechanical sources of pain such as pressure from the fetal presenting part (Fig. 3.26). In addition the weight of the pregnant uterus at term, pressing on the

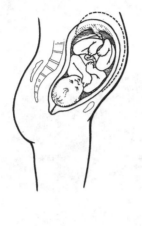
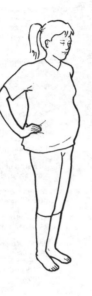

A

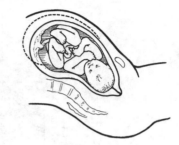

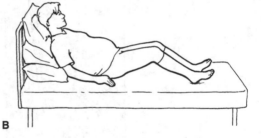

B

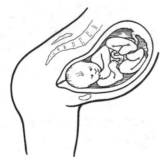

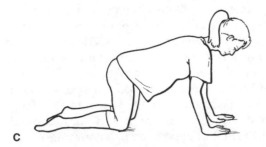

C

Figure 3.26 The potential effect of gravity on uterine action. **A** During labour the uterus contracts and tilts forwards. The resistance to gravity is naturally minimised in the upright position. **B** When labouring in the semi-reclining position, contractions work against the natural force of gravity. **C** When kneeling or leaning forwards, contraction of the uterus meets least resistance.

inferior vena cava when the woman is flat on her back, will in itself reduce venous return and cardiac output, ultimately potentially causing fetal distress.

Caldeyro-Barcia (1979) described the positions women spontaneously adopt throughout normal labour. These include sitting, walking, kneeling, standing and leaning forwards (Fig. 3.27). It has to be assumed that women will spontaneously change their position in order to attempt to reduce pain; at the same time any position which is naturally maintained will indicate that the woman is experiencing a degree of comfort. Midwives will sometimes encourage a woman to change her position if it looks as though it may be uncomfortable. Women will not usually put

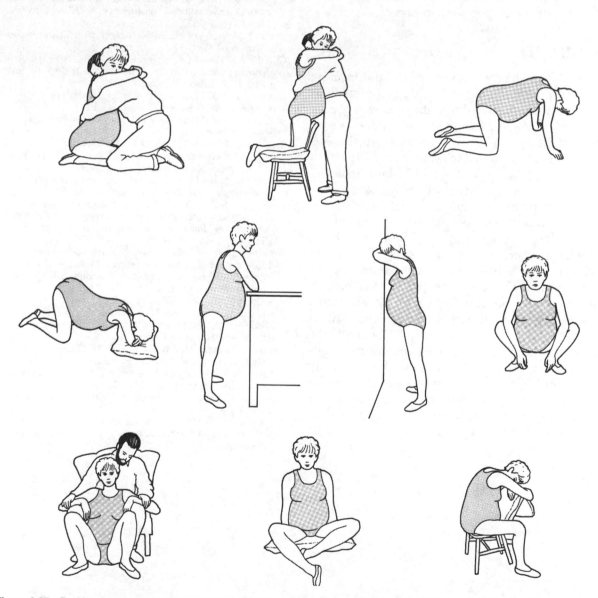

Figure 3.27   Positions women may adopt to effectively relieve pain in labour (reproduced with kind permission from Bevis 1989).

themselves into a more painful position, even if it looks that way to the observer. Melzack et al (1991) investigated the effect of maternal position on labour pain. This study suggested that women experienced significantly less pain, particularly back pain, when in a vertical position than when they were horizontal. It has become apparent in recent years that many women have been encouraged to labour in a position that is convenient for the midwife or the doctor in attendance rather than for the labouring woman herself.

SUMMARY

The midwife has an important role in informing and supporting the woman throughout labour. It is through her knowledge of the processes of pain transmission and perception, modulation of pain and methods of relieving pain in labour that she will enable the woman to achieve a positive birth experience. For some this will be best achieved by using modern forms of analgesia such as Entonox, pethidine and epidural anaesthesia. These women will benefit from experiencing what they perceive as a 'pain-free' labour. However, there are an increasing number of women who believe that taking control of the birth and having responsibility for the process also provides an equally rewarding emotional experience through a sense of achievement. It is the midwife's responsibility to be with the woman and to know her well enough to understand her real needs. This can only be effectively achieved by being with the woman throughout labour, ideally by having met her before labour begins and discussing her needs with her, and by the continuing use of good communication skills at all times.

REFERENCES

Balaskas J 1991 New active birth, revised edn. Thorsons, London

Bevis R 1989 Pain relief and comfort in labour. In: Bennett V R, Brown L K (eds) Myles textbook for midwives, 11th edn. Churchill Livingstone, Edinburgh, p 177–191

Bonica J 1994 Labour pain. In: Wall P, Melzack R (eds) Textbook of pain. Churchill Livingstone, Edinburgh, p 615–641

Caldeyro-Barcia R 1979 The influence of maternal position on time of spontaneous rupture of the membranes, progress of labour and fetal head compression, Birth and the Family Journal 6 (1): 7–15

Clancy J, McVicar A 1992 Subjectivity of pain. British Journal of Nursing, 1 (1): 8–12

Gintzler A R, Peters L C, Karnisarvk B R 1983 Attenuation of pregnancy-induced analgesia by hypogastric neurectomy in rats. Brain Research 277: 186–188

Guyton A C 1987 Basic neuroscience: anatomy and physiology. W. B. Saunders, Philadelphia

Melzack R, Wall P 1988 The challenge of pain. Penguin Books, London

Melzack R, Belanger E, Lacroix R 1991 Labour pain: effect of maternal position on front and back pain. Journal of Pain and Symptom Management 6 (8): 476–480

Polden M, Mantle J 1992 Physiotherapy in obstetrics and gynaecology. Butterworth Heinemann, Oxford

Rutishauser S 1994 Physiology and anatomy: a basis for nursing and health care. Churchill Livingstone, Edinburgh

Sagaday M 1995 Renewing our faith in second stage. Midwifery Today 33: 29–43

Simkins P 1989 Non-pharmacological methods of pain relief during labour. In: Chalmers I, Enkin M, Keirse M J N C (eds) Effective care in pregnancy and childbirth. Oxford University Press, Oxford, p 893–912

The Open University 1991 Module B1: neuronal structure and function. The Open University, Milton Keynes

Thibodeau G A 1992 Structure and function of the body, 9th edn. Mosby Year Books, London

Varassi G, Bazzano C, Edwards W T 1989 Effects of physical activity on maternal plasma beta-endorphin levels and perception of labour pain, American Journal of Obstetrics and Gynaecology 160 (3): 707–712

Voke J 1986 Transmitting the right signals. Nursing Times, Sept 24, p 47–49

Weisenberg M 1994 Cognitive aspects of pain. In: Wall P, Melzack R (eds) Textbook of pain. Churchill Livingstone, Edinburgh, p 275–289

4

Psychology of pain in labour

Sue Moore

LEARNING OUTCOMES

At the end of this chapter the reader will have

- **identified some of the main psychological factors influencing pain perception in labour**

- **considered the effect of midwifery care on the perception of pain**

- **identified some factors associated with the psychological modulation of pain in labour**

- **an introduction to psychological explanations relating to individual differences which may influence pain perception and control.**

Psychological and anthropological studies have shown that pain is not simply a function of the amount of bodily damage alone. Rather the amount and quality of pain we feel are determined by our previous experiences and how well we remember them, by our ability to understand the cause of pain and to grasp its consequences. Even the culture in which we have been brought up plays an essential role in how we feel and respond to pain

(Melzack & Wall 1988).

The above paragraph demonstrates some of the main features relating to the psychology of pain. Psychology traditionally examines the many facets of human thought, emotion and experience which influence how people react in a given situation. Psychological factors associated with pain perception and experience are therefore important for understanding how people cope with pain and what forms of pain relief are likely to be most beneficial for each person, especially for the relief of labour pain. This chapter will therefore examine some of the subjective, emotional and cognitive aspects of pain in labour, together with some of the factors which influence pain perception.

It is frequently said that pain is a subjective experience. Human beings are unique individuals, each person perceiving, experiencing and responding to pain in their own unique way. The emotional aspect of pain is a feature of many psychological issues relating to the pain experience. Emotions associated with pain include feelings of anger, fear, anxiety and guilt, and may even include sexual arousal (Craig 1994). It is often the emotional component of pain that is 'transferred' to those who care for individuals experiencing pain. A woman who is afraid or angry in labour will communicate her distress more readily and those supporting her will frequently reflect the emotions she feels, often unknowingly. Such factors add to the complexity of the psychological elements associated with pain in labour.

Emotional events surrounding pain are further influenced by each person's cognitive appraisal of the painful event. Cognition involves the mental processes of knowing, perceiving, imagining, judging and reasoning (Weisenberg 1994). There are individuals who will 'catastrophise' by a process of negative thinking and ideas, often making negative statements about themselves (Craig 1994). Methods for dealing with negative thinking include stress-inoculation training and distraction techniques, which can be effective in relieving pain. Stress-inoculation training usually involves a detailed programme through which the individual can identify the cause of their negative thinking, and then identify and carry out specific methods for dealing with the situation as it arises. This technique has been particularly effective in stress and anger management, yet has also proved beneficial for pain management. Other techniques, which include relaxation and hypnosis, are believed to reduce anxiety and relieve tension, and consequently to enhance feelings of self-efficacy (Keefe et al 1986). The cognitive component of pain is therefore relevant to each person's ability to cope with pain, and because of this, many techniques for reducing pain are based on the knowledge of individual cognitive processes.

The behavioural approach to psychology lays emphasis on the belief that individuals learn behaviour from their social environment, and that people are conditioned to behave as they do through forms of reward or punishment (the 'carrot and stick' principle). It is perhaps because childbirth for many women brings its own 'reward' that labour pain is often perceived as a positive experience (see p. 11). Cognitive–behavioural techniques are used effectively in clinical practice by psychologists and psychiatrists to deal with many psychological aspects of human experience, to help an individual to recognise and manage negative thought processes by a process of training and development of skills and coping strategies.

PAIN BEHAVIOUR

In psychological terms, it is each person's emotions and thought processes which, together with previous experience, will influence how they behave when in pain. Turk et al (1985) identified that people generally respond to pain with certain facial and audible expressions of distress, typically displayed as the clenching of teeth, grimacing and moaning. Distorted posture is also typical, as is walking in a guarded manner, stooping and holding the painful area. Displays of emotion such as irritability and the adoption of a 'sick role' are characteristic behaviour patterns which accompany pain. As a result of these patterns, individuals then receive care and attention from others, which in turn reinforces the pain behaviour. It has been suggested that pain can be used manipulatively, for example to elicit advantages such as social support, to control relatives or to avoid intimacy (Latham 1988). Some people may consequently mimic pain behaviour to feign illness. It is possible, then, that if a person is labelled as manipulative, her level of pain may be underestimated or even disregarded by some professionals.

Pain behaviour during labour

Most midwives will readily recognise pain behaviour associated with labour, since it is very characteristic, and the experienced midwife will usually be able to assess the stage of labour based entirely on the woman's behaviour pattern. Robertson (1994) documented some of these patterns of behaviour as they occur in normal labour:

- pre-labour
  —'nesting' and spurts of energy
  —intuitive feelings, recognising subtle body changes
- early labour
  —excitement, and anticipation, restlessness and nervousness
  —wanting to walk about, making conversation, making eye contact, needing companionship and distraction
- established labour
  —avoids conversation, rests quietly between contractions
  —becomes passive
  —finds own position, often sitting, head resting on arms
  —needing non-disruptive support from birth companions
  —develops her own pattern of breathing
- transition
  —sudden changes take place
  —feels out of control, unable to cope, 'wanting to go home'
  —restless, moving around
  —irrational comments, often angry with birth companion
  —verbalising, sometimes screaming
- second stage
  —becomes calmer, 'second wind'
  —a sense of purpose takes over, intense concentration
  —feels and looks calmer.

The experienced midwife will have regularly observed these behaviour patterns, and will encourage the woman to be aware of what is happening so that she can anticipate and develop appropriate coping strategies. She will also reassure the woman by encouraging her to not feel embarrassed or humiliated by what she is doing or saying. It appears that pain behaviour associated with labour is somewhat different to types of behaviour associated with acute and chronic pain. In normal labour there is a very distinct pattern, which does not conform so readily to the 'sick role' behaviour.

In a study analysing vocalisations made by women in labour, Baker & Kenner (1993) suggested that a greater sensitivity to these sounds will reduce the amount of intervention, typically vaginal examinations, during labour. Every midwife will be familiar with this concept and will be able to recognise progress in labour as displayed by such vocalisations, particularly the onset of transition and, even more specifically, the onset of the second stage of labour. Increased sensitivity to pain behaviour is therefore one of the skills of midwifery practice.

LABOUR ENVIRONMENT

Behaviour associated with pain in labour is often considered unacceptable by those surrounding the labouring woman, because they find her vocalisation uncomfortable, disquieting and even embarrassing; this can lead to a belief that it should be reduced as soon as possible. This often means that the woman is encouraged to have sedation, usually by administration of narcotic agents such as pethidine. Pain relief is therefore sometimes encouraged not to reduce the woman's pain, but merely to comfort those who are observing.

Robertson (1994) suggests that 'a basic belief in women's ability to give birth, unassisted, is at the centre of the empowerment process'. This does not mean that pharmacological analgesia should be withheld, but that an environment suitable for a labouring woman should be made available. The 'environment' is usually regarded as the birthing room, together with its fixtures and fittings. Although these things are significant in helping a woman to cope psychologically with labour, it is the 'emotional environment' that is considered to be most relevant. A positive emotional environment that helps a woman to feel relaxed, calm and confident can only be provided by those giving support and care throughout her labour.

The typical labour ward environment, however, does not lend itself to the privacy and tranquillity that women normally need. Usually designed as a 'clinical' environment, it demonstrates the features of many accident and emergency departments—

i.e. it is designed for carrying out clinical procedures easily and effectively, and not to provide a natural birthing environment. As maternity services became hospitalised and centralised in the 1970s, little consideration appears to have been given to the environmental needs of the woman in childbirth. A natural acceptance of medicalised environments alongside medicalised care appears to have developed. Midwives and maternity services personnel have over recent years spent much time, money and effort converting clinical environments, usually by adding furniture and fittings to create more 'homely' surroundings. The Department of Health has now acknowledged that a labouring woman has special environmental needs and one can only hope that future designs of maternity units will do the same:

The environment in which birth takes place is important to a woman and her partner, and it should be as supportive and comfortable as possible. If the birth takes place in hospital, the beds in the delivery suites should be comfortable for the woman, and she should be free to move around and adopt new positions as labour progresses

(Department of Health 1993).

METHODS OF PAIN RELIEF IN LABOUR

Expectations of pain-relieving methods and attitudes towards pain relief have changed a great deal over the last century. Attitudes formed from society's belief that pain, especially pain in labour, was a consequence of original sin, and from beliefs based on religious dogma, began to change as a new scientific era and period of medical development gave rise to a belief in scientific and causal explanations for human ills, together with the general belief that medical science was able to treat such ills.

Traditionally, methods of pain relief have been regarded as limited, particularly for reducing pain in labour. It was not until 1853 that the discovery of ether by James Young Simpson, and the subsequent use of chloroform by Queen Victoria, heralded the beginning of obstetric anaesthesia and analgesia. It is of interest to note that this coincided with a rise in the involvement of medical men in midwifery (Donnison 1988). Moir (1986) decries the fact that:

Until 1847 there had been no really effective methods of anaesthesia or analgesia. From Ancient Babylonian times attempts had been made to relieve the pains of labour and delivery but these can have met with little success. Any success probably depended more on faith than on pharmacological efficacy and most methods could be broadly classified as psychological ...

And yet a survey conducted by the National Birthday Trust of women giving birth during one week in 1990 (Chamberlain et al 1993) identified that women, in assessing the effectiveness of the current methods of pain relief, found relaxation and massage no less effective than the commonly used pharmacological analgesics such as Entonox (50% nitrous oxide and 50% oxygen) or pethidine. Data from over 10 000 women undergoing birth were included in this study. Of the sample population, 27% believed pethidine to be very good for relieving their labour pain, 18% thought it was poor, and 11% found it to be of no use at all. On the other hand, 35% of the population found relaxation to be effective, while only 9% thought that it had a poor effect, and 3% found it to be of no use at all. It would of course be rash to make generalisations using such data, however there appears to be a distinct need to examine such evidence further. Pharmacological methods of pain relief may be seen as modern medicine's version of chloroform in childbirth, however it would appear that non-pharmacological methods have the potential to be at least as effective as modern analgesia. Modern methods of pain relief in labour therefore perpetuate the myth that medicine is a panacea. The modern tradition within midwifery practice has been to assess at what time the woman needs drugs during her labour; the issue would appear to be whether she is enabled to select a method of pain relief, pharmacological or non-pharmacological, which is appropriate to her individual needs.

The ideal method of pain relief in labour has been described by Lewis & Chamberlain (1990) as 'not harming the mother or fetus ... and does not interfere with uterine action, does not lead to more operative intervention or depress the respiratory system of the newborn; and its effect should be easy to administer, foolproof, and predictable and constant in its effects'. Paradoxically, it is pharmacological methods such as pethidine, inhalation analgesia and epidural anaesthesia which are then identified as the ideal forms of pain relief in labour. Such methods may not necessarily be 'easy to administer'—pethidine is given by intramuscular injection and is a 'controlled drug' with associated legislation for prescribing, storage and administration; an epidural is an anaesthetic procedure and as such can only be performed by an experienced anaesthetist, and is also associated with long-term morbidity (MacArthur et al 1990); finally, Entonox is an inhalation analgesic which, although the woman is able to control administration herself, is still a drug and therefore again has implications for storage and prescribing. Although these pharmacological methods are to some extent predictable in their action on most occasions, there are always possible side-effects for both mother and fetus in labour (British Medical Association and Royal Pharmaceutical Society 1994).

Errors in administration of drugs are an aspect of practice of which every professional involved in any form of medical care must be aware. Although statistical evidence is not readily available concerning the numbers of individuals involved in legislative and disciplinary proceedings due to drug-related errors, there is no doubt that such incidents do occur. It is therefore difficult to consider pharmacological methods of pain relief as 'foolproof'. Dickersin (1989) identified some of the potential effects of drugs used for pain relief in labour, such as respiratory depression of mother and neonate, and possible long-term neurological problems; it would appear therefore that psychological methods are arguably the only means of fulfilling the criteria for 'ideal' forms of pain relief.

PSYCHOLOGY, PREGNANCY, CHILDBIRTH AND MIDWIFERY CARE

Beliefs about childbirth

Childbirth is traditionally recognised by many psychologists as a time of increased anxiety, a 'period of crisis involving profound psychological changes' (Bibring 1959), or a major life transition. However, childbirth may also be seen as a natural occurrence in the procreation of the human species: 'pregnancy, childbirth and motherhood are an intrinsic part of women's experience' (Ussher 1989). As such, there is a tension between the views of pregnancy as a life crisis and pregnancy as a natural physiological and psychological process—i.e. part of life's progression; a life event; a normative transition (Kimmel 1980). This debate may be extended by considering the assumptions on which maternity care is founded, as well as the implementation of such care for women during pregnancy and childbirth.

The experience of pregnancy and childbirth is inevitably influenced by the type of care provided within the maternity services. Whether pregnancy is viewed as a period to be 'managed', whereby women are perceived as needing the facilities made available by modern science and the technological advances of the era, or whether it is perceived as a time at which women need the support of their peers, family and social networks to enable acceptance and normalisation of the event, will depend on the view taken by society at the time in question. Women describe childbirth as a momentous event; as a time of transformation; as unique; and as a period when emotional and spiritual aspects of their lives become some of their prime concerns (Page 1988). Page recognised that one of the main principles of care for women in childbirth should be to treat birth as 'more than a medical event …'.

Obstetric services currently emphasise the need to detect and diagnose the possible complications with which women may be confronted during childbirth. The potential for over-diagnosis and other iatrogenic effects, as well as increased rates of medical intervention, is inevitably increased. There are some authors who suggest that active management, such as the induction of labour, leads to the increased use of pharmacological analgesia, as well as increased rates of forceps delivery, Caesarean section, and the admission of neonates to intensive care baby units (Kitzinger 1991, Cartwright 1979). Such interventions will inevitably increase the experience of pain associated with childbirth. The perception of pain may therefore be influenced by medical events which are potentially avoidable. Some people argue that women's apparent acceptance of pharmacological methods of pain relief may, in fact, be associated with the increased medicalisation and intervention associated with modern childbirth practices.

Psychological views

Psychologists also focus on aspects predicting pathology, such as postnatal depression, puerperal psychosis, parenting dysfunction and other disorders, rather than exploring and understanding the actual birth experience. Current frameworks for midwifery practice are based on beliefs that care is individualised, acknowledging a woman's physical, social, educational, spiritual and psychological needs. A knowledge of some of the individual psychological factors associated with pain and pain relief in labour will potentially increase understanding and appreciation of the uniqueness of the birth experience for women, thereby acknowledging the emotional and spiritual aspects. Feminist writers like Ussher (1989) question the dearth of discussion relating to the female body and reproductive issues; she suggests that it is '… part of the practice which ignores experiences which are peculiar to women …'

Women's experiences, feelings and concerns in pregnancy were investigated by Combes & Schonveld (1992). They showed that what particularly preoccupied women at various stages throughout pregnancy were anxieties about labour, particularly whether they would know if labour had started and how painful it was going to be. The women surveyed felt that these were issues for which they did not always receive adequate or appropriate information from professionals, including midwives. Passing on information is an aspect of midwifery practice which in the past has been found wanting (Kirkham 1989). Kirkham's descriptive, observational study illustrates how the use of language and medical jargon, communication blocking styles, the hierarchical service and the birth setting can influence the type of care women receive during labour and how they perceive the care. As Kirkham stated, midwifery could re-establish its autonomy by developing its body of knowledge. An understanding of the psychological processes associated with the experience of pain in labour would inform practice, thus increasing knowledge relating to the emotional experience of childbirth, and also improving the psychological and social well-being of women and their families, as well as identifying any possible or actual pathological consequences. In this way, the true needs of women at this most significant life transition would be identified and met.

There is no doubt that labour is a painful process. However, the perception of pain intensity and unpleasantness is often associated with, and potentiated by, many other factors. Labour pain has physiological and emotional components which make it more difficult to evaluate the experience of birth. It is therefore important not only to consider the various methods of pain relief, pharmacological or otherwise, which may influence a woman's expectation of labour, but also to examine those factors which may have an influence on the birthing process and which are therefore likely to affect a woman's overall experience.

PSYCHOLOGICAL FACTORS ASSOCIATED WITH PAIN PERCEPTION IN LABOUR

As outlined in Chapter 2, there have been many attempts over the years to explain the meaning of pain and pain perception. These attempts serve to illustrate the intricacies of pain, which is subjective in nature, and necessarily includes anatomical, physiological, psychological and social components. Pain is considered to be multidimensional, consisting of sensory-discriminative, cognitive-evaluative and affective-motivational dimensions (Melzack & Wall 1988). Mountcastle (1980), for example, described pain as 'that sensory experience evoked by stimuli that injure or threaten to destroy tissue, defined introspectively by man as that which hurts'. Labour pain, however, may be seen as a unique form of pain which is not directly the consequence of injury. Although injury may be incurred in the process of labour, it can be argued that such injury is more likely to occur as a result of intervention rather than as a consequence of normal labour. Such interventions include the use of oxytocic drugs in labour to increase uterine activity, or the indiscriminate use of episiotomy, and are therefore the source of less acceptable 'hurt'.

A woman's discomfort in labour may then be further potentiated by postures which reduce the effectiveness of normal physiological processes for birth. The transition to birth in hospital, and arguably the accompanying sick role, has led to women in labour being encouraged to lie flat on their backs to give birth. It has been argued that this may ultimately increase intervention rates, and consequently increase levels of pain experienced in labour (Inch 1982). One can see, therefore, that there are many factors—physical, psychological, social and environmental—which influence the perception of pain, and which cannot readily be isolated from the total childbearing experience.

Feelings of 'control'

Various psychological factors have been shown to influence a woman's perception of pain and her ability to cope with it. Positive or negative feelings about the labour experience would appear, in many instances, to relate to whether the woman feels in control of events. Such events often relate to labour outcome, that is whether the birth process is perceived as a satisfying experience, and whether the woman feels that she has had control over decision-making at all times. Studies relating to personal control in childbirth present some complex findings. As illustrated by psychological theories relating to locus of control (Rotter 1966), when examined at an individual level, 'control' means different things to different people. Rotter's theory examines the extent to which people see themselves (internal locus), or other people and influences external to the individual (external locus), as being in control of any given set of events. Many difficulties are encountered when concepts such as 'internal locus' and 'external locus' of control are applied to childbearing. Women may experience little control over events, since control is frequently maintained by professionals who 'manage' labour. The degree of autonomy which a woman has throughout birth will often be influenced by those in attendance during the event, and also by the woman's own belief systems and ability to control events.

Niven (1994) found that women's perceptions of control related to a variety of aspects of labour and birth. For some, control was concerned with the duration of labour, while for others it was participation in decisions relating to the management of the labour and delivery, such as choice of analgesia. Others saw being 'out of control' as 'showing themselves up'. A study by Scott-Palmer & Skevington (1981) demonstrated that women with an internal locus of control experienced higher levels of pain in labour than those with an external locus of control. Such findings suggest that an internal locus of control—feeling 'in control'—may not be advantageous, even though a high internal locus of control is often associated with indicators of good psychological health (Phares 1976). Some people argue that women often believe it is more acceptable to leave the decision-making to the midwife. Midwives in turn see their role as being the woman's advocate, enabling her to make appropriate, informed choices.

Niven (1994) found that 'trusting the staff' was associated with significantly lower levels of pain in labour; however there were some relationships between 'trusting the staff' and the need for analgesia, such as Entonox and pethidine, which were administered by the staff. This study highlights the importance of the midwife's role in encouraging and supporting women in their use of relaxation and coping strategies, which in turn give the woman a sense of achievement. Those women who had a good relationship with the staff were able to use a greater number of coping strategies. However, there was some suggestion that midwives' attitudes towards certain coping techniques was sometimes 'hostile', particularly those strategies that are termed 'NCT type'.

Although this study was not generally representative of midwives' attitudes towards the use of coping techniques by women in labour, there is some suggestion that staff sometimes lack confidence in a woman's ability to cope with labour. Some midwives have a fundamental belief that pharmacological methods are the only effective form of analgesia, and are therefore likely to promote them more readily. Niven also found that 'trusting the staff' was significantly associated with attendance at antenatal preparation classes.

Preparation for childbirth

The influence of childbirth preparation classes on the perception and modulation of pain in labour has been acknowledged for many years. Melzack & Wall (1988) reviewed the evidence relating to the effects of prepared childbirth training, acknowledging the methods of Dick Read (1942) and Lamaze (1970). A study conducted by Melzack et al (1981) demonstrated that prepared childbirth training decreased pain by reducing fear and anxiety. Melzack found that the effectiveness of antenatal preparation is also influenced by the person presenting the classes. For example, a correlation was found between the pain experienced by women during childbirth and the enthusiasm of their instructor.

Skevington & Wilkes (1992) found that the type of childbirth preparation class was inclined to influence a woman's belief in pain control. In their study, women attending 'birthing centre' classes were committed to natural childbirth and had weak beliefs in the power of doctors to control their labour pain. It is possible that a woman's beliefs surrounding the birth process, particularly as to whether the birth is a natural or medically managed event, will influence the eventual outcome. Skevington & Wilkes reported that women who attended the birthing centre class had a higher internal locus of control than women attending National Health Service (NHS) classes run at local hospitals. They also found that some women who attended classes outside of the NHS showed less evidence of depressive symptoms, particularly in the postnatal period. These factors indicate the significance of the content of childbirth preparation classes, where they are presented and who presents them.

Many childbirth preparation classes introduce women and their birth partners to the management of pain in labour in two ways—there are relaxation classes and there are usually one or two sessions on methods of pain relief, sometimes involving an anaesthetist. Combes & Schonveld (1992) indicated in their review of parent education that 'very little attention has been paid as to whether women actually use the pain control techniques they have been taught' in preparation for labour. This study identified that midwives and other health professionals need to consider the appropriateness of all classes to individual needs, as well as considering their educational quality, especially in terms of their reality to the actual situation. Emphasis is usually placed on introducing certain relaxation techniques, but often without evaluating the effectiveness for the client group. Effective preparation may be achieved by teaching women in small groups; identifying individual coping strategies for labour; and ensuring that the teacher is a midwife with whom the pregnant women have established a trusting relationship.

Anxiety

As Combes & Schonveld (1992) found, negative feelings surrounding the perception of pain in labour are often associated with anxiety during pregnancy. Reading & Cox (1985) found that, in particular, anxiety occurring after 32 weeks of pregnancy was a predictor of pain in labour. In addition, Reading & Cox subsequently found that pain in labour was a predictor of postpartum mood. The explanations for such findings are potentially manifold, but negative feelings during pregnancy, which could then be associated with the perception of pain in labour, must be considered. In turn, the possibility of such emotional turmoil creating psychological problems within the mothering role must be acknowledged. Robson & Kumar (1980) found that severe pain experienced in labour can inhibit maternal emotions towards the baby. The recognition that events during the childbearing process can have a detrimental effect on parent–infant attachment, and on the subsequent parental relationship, is also reported in Bowlby (1969) and Condon (1993). This has been found to be especially true if an exhausting, pain-filled labour leads to prolonged separation between mother and infant in the immediate postnatal period.

COPING STRATEGIES AND THE EFFECT OF CARERS

It is important to identify methods of pain modulation which optimise the birth experience, and thus improve mother–infant interaction in the immediate postnatal period. Niven (1994) examined the role played by psychological factors in modulating pain perception in labour; she considered such things as relaxation and breathing techniques, distraction, imagery, reversal of affect, normalization of pain and idiosyncratic strategies. The use of imagery includes techniques such as imagining how the baby will look when it's born, or imagining sun-filled beach holidays. Reversal of affect is a strategy whereby women respond positively to the pain, seeing it as a sign of progress in labour. Those women who 'normalised' pain perceived it as a normal part of labour. Those who used idiosyncratic techniques included a 'concert pianist who played symphonies in her head during labour, and a policewoman who thought about the agony that some accident victims must have felt …'. Such individualised coping strategies would seem to indicate that some women have within themselves certain characteristics which enable them to deal with pain in very specific ways.

Niven also asked the midwives to complete an assessment of women's pain experience. Although midwives' assessment of the pain correlated highly with that experienced by the women in the study (both groups perceived labour as painful), the actual score recorded by the midwives was consistently lower than that recorded by the women. The variation in pain perception between women undergoing childbirth and the professionals caring for them was also demonstrated by Rajan (1993). It was shown that professionals, including midwives and medical staff, were more likely to agree with each other about the effectiveness of pain relief received by women than they were to agree with the women themselves, and were less likely to respond to those women who believed their pain relief was poor.

As Niven suggests, as yet there is little known about the interactive dynamics experienced in the relationship between a midwife and the woman for whom she is caring. An American study (Mackey & Stepans 1994) identified those qualities of the 'labour-nurse' perceived as favourable by the women in labour. These nurses were evaluated favourably because of positive participation, acceptance, information giving, encouragement, presence and competence. Although midwifery practice in the UK is very different from the role of the American obstetric nurse, it can be argued that emotional support in terms of the characteristics and behaviour of the nurse or midwife is a common feature within both roles. O'Driscoll & Meagher (1980) emphasised that support in labour was more than a presence, and recognised that student midwives, who were often the person continuously providing support for women in labour, used interactional skills such as eye contact, touch and rapport. These skills are arguably the manifestations of interpersonal behaviour which itself increases reassurance, reduces anxiety and thereby potentially reduces pain sensation. The importance of certain qualities attributed to the person supporting labouring women is therefore acknowledged. 'Being cared for in labour by a midwife whom she knows may be reassuring to a woman and reduce her need for pharmacological pain relief' (Department of Health 1993).

Social support

In many developing countries, women are attended in childbirth by traditional birth attendants, often family members such as the mother, mother-in-law or sisters. There are women within such societies who are 'experts' in supporting women throughout labour, providing 'comfort techniques and ways of assisting birth by transforming the woman's psychological state …' (Kitzinger 1991). Hospitalisation during childbirth in industrialised societies has been recognised as causing separation of women from family members, implementation of rigid procedures and lack of choice in labour (Keirse et al 1989).

Typically, the effect of having family members present during labour and birth, as a means of social support, on the reduction of labour pain has been studied in relation to the presence of husbands. Niven (1985) found that women who were accompanied by their husbands during labour judged their presence to be helpful. It was demonstrated that the woman's overall perception of 'helpfulness' was influential in the reported modulation of pain; a helpful husband was one whose presence was 'comforting', because he was 'someone familiar' and 'someone to hold on to', both metaphorically and physically.

Whereas it was at one time traditional for men to pace the hospital waiting room floor during childbirth, the current practice is for them to be present for the labour and throughout the birth of their baby. However, this new approach, although welcome, can give rise to certain dilemmas. Although the majority of men want to be present at the birth and are pleased to be involved (Macmillan 1995), there is a suggestion that for some men, being present at the birth has an adverse effect on the couple's longer term relationship, particularly their sexual relationship (O'Driscoll 1994). Thus, it appears that the complexities associated with pain relief in labour are accentuated, as the emotional cost impinges on the potential well-being of the couple's relationship. Interestingly, there is a current resurgence of female family members and friends supporting women in the labour ward, a factor which has been subject to little evaluation.

Individual differences

Midwifery is a practice based profession and midwives have traditionally developed their perceptions and beliefs from the art of being 'with woman' (direct translation of the Anglo-Saxon word 'midwife'). This partnership usually develops from a relationship built up over time and encompasses the intuitive, caring skills of the expert practitioner, thus providing both physical and emotional support for the woman in labour. The art of midwifery is therefore founded on a tradition of observation, interaction and empathy, caring and supporting a woman in a state of physical well-being, throughout an emotionally demanding time. Traditionally midwives in their clinical practice may have therefore adopted common-sense perceptions of certain groups of women, which would have resulted in the initiation of generalisations about the individual and created certain stereotypes. Although observations can be a rich source of evidence for experiences in childbirth, criticism of the intuitive approach to practice may be justified if observations and judgments are based on generalisations and assumptions which are prejudicial to the woman in pregnancy and labour. This is one reason for the current research approach to practice which is based on a scientific tradition of objective study ensuring that care is appropriate, generalisations are reliable and theories are validated.

In everyday experience, it is not unusual for people to be classified in terms of their personal characteristics, whereby many generalisations and assumptions about individuals are made. Women with different personal characteristics will identify distinct needs, especially in labour. There are instances in midwifery practice whereby women with specific idiosyncratic thoughts and ideas about how they expect their pregnancy and labour to progress, are viewed in a stereotypical way.

Stereotypes encompass attitudes and beliefs about specific groups, which may be unfavourable and derogatory, and can therefore be identified as prejudicial, for example, homeless people are all criminals, women who take drugs are all prostitutes. If such prejudicial thoughts are apparent in behaviour (i.e. the thoughts are 'acted out'), it becomes discrimination. Stereotyping and prejudice are more likely if the person is less well known. Prejudice can therefore often be overcome if the individuals concerned build up a closeness, by working together and sharing common goals.

An example of some of the common stereotypes made by midwives was studied by Green et al (1990) and described how women were often seen as the 'well-educated, middle-class, NCT (National Childbirth Trust) type' or the 'uneducated, working-class type'. A woman who is knowledgeable, articulate and assertive, who enters the maternity services with a clear idea of how her pregnancy and labour will be managed, ideally anticipating a natural, drug-free labour, and likely to attend childbirth preparation classes both privately and within the NHS, may well be perceived as the 'well-educated, middle-class, NCT type'. Alternatively, a 'compliant' woman, who has no perception of any facility other than the routine, medicalised maternity service, who is not very articulate, and therefore not able to question the form of maternity care with which she is presented, may be seen as 'the uneducated, working-class type'. Green's study demonstrated that the former stereotypes were often inaccurate, particularly the belief that the 'NCT type' is more likely to want to avoid the use of drugs in labour. In fact, dealing with the stereotype of the working-class woman, they stated that 'far from being unconcerned with birth as a fulfilling experience it was as important to her as it was for the more educated and middle-class woman ...' and that she 'was far from abdicating all responsibilities to the staff'.

Green et al went on to explore the subjects' perceptions of pain relief in labour in relation to educational and social backgrounds. It was demonstrated that those women who were classified as well educated were more committed to a drug-free labour than other women, but then they were also more informed about the side-effects of specific pain-relieving drugs. The study also suggested that less well educated women had relatively greater expectations of birth as a fulfilling experience, contradicting the common perception of many professionals that working-class women don't want to know or aren't interested in what happens to them. However, in Green et al's study, less well educated women believed that they would have less involvement and control over events, an expectation which was to a large extent found to be justified. Quine et al (1993) found that working-class women felt less prepared for birth, and were less satisfied with the information they were given, as well as with the birth experience. The working-class women in this study were particularly worried about the pain of childbirth and how to cope with it, but many were inhibited from discussing their

anxieties in front of more 'articulate middle-class women'. It is clear, therefore, that women's expectations are immersed in many sociological factors, particularly levels of education, but also age, class and their ability to control events. The need to explore these issues further in relation to the implementation of midwifery care is apparent, particularly if attitudes towards the varying groups create unwanted stereotypes and lead to possible prejudice and discrimination.

Variations in individual pain perception and levels of satisfaction with the birth experience are influenced by sociological as well as psychological factors, all of which add to the complexity of understanding. Midwives, as the prime carers, identify the importance of providing individualised care. Current philosophies of midwifery care contend that the childbearing woman is 'an individual' and that, as such, her individual needs must be recognised. It is therefore important to understand whether those characteristics which differentiate individuals, such as aspects of personality, are predictors for the perception of pain in labour and thus potentially for satisfaction with the birth experience.

Traditionally, psychology has attempted to explain consistencies in behaviour by developing some well known theories relating to personality. Characteristics unique to every individual can make their experience of the world different, as well as affecting the way in which each person views others, and moreover the way individuals see themselves. Eysenck (1953) developed a well known typology by categorising individuals with certain internal characteristics as conforming to particular points on what were termed extraversion–introversion and neuroticism–stability dimensions. Another example is that of Allport (1937), who developed a trait personality theory as a response to and reaction against Freud's psychodynamic theory which was prevalent at that time. Allport (1961) proposed that individuals are the product of their genetic make-up and of social learning. In contrast to psychodynamics, he believed that individuals' characteristics were a product of conscious self-directed mental processes. However, the psychodynamic tradition reflected in the pschoanalytic theories of Freud,

Adler and Jung (the latter incidentally having proposed an introversion–extraversion typology) focuses on personality as a development of characteristics seated in the processes of the unconscious mind. Currently the pschoanalytic tradition in relation to mothering, pregnancy and childbirth is presented by the work of Raphael-Leff. In true psychoanalytic convention, Raphael-Leff's (1983) theory relating to specific unconscious and conscious processes in pregnancy and motherhood was based on clinical experience as a psychoanalyst. The following section will explore the application of Raphael-Leff's model to women's experience of pain and pain relief in labour.

PSYCHOANALYSIS AND CHILDBIRTH

Raphael-Leff based her theory on assumptions founded in the Freudian tradition of ego-psychology, emphasising the infant's physiological needs and 'anaclictic type attachment to the mother', and the object relations school which views the infant as a social being. Raphael-Leff acknowledged that such views were presented from the perspective of the infant rather than the mother, and proposed that maternal responses are 'adherent in the *unconscious* orientation of different types of mothers to their babies …' (my italics). A model which identified two specific 'orientations' to mothering based on these assumptions was subsequently devised:

- The 'Regulator' mother regards her baby as 'a bundle of needs'; pregnancy as an 'emotional upheaval' when personal identity is threatened; labour as 'depleting', a 'medical event', 'inflicted pain'; and the ideal birth as being 'civilised' with analgesia and monitoring. She must regulate gratification of the baby's needs, training the baby and making him/her 'adapt to environmental reality'.
- The 'Facilitator' mother regards the baby as 'an intimate from birth or pregnancy'; pregnancy as a time of heightened emotional experience when personal identity is enhanced; labour as 'exhilarating', 'an intimate event'; and the ideal birth as natural, resisting all pharmacological and

technological interventions. To facilitate the baby's needs she must adapt to him/her.

This model may explain some of the stereotypical views held by midwives in relation to women's perceptions of pregnancy and labour, as identified previously. Raphael-Leff (1991) in fact suggests that 'the main value of this model is to make sense of confusing and seeming contradictory patterns, where in their demand of professionals, some women appear to want just the opposite to other women'. In later work, Raphael-Leff (1993) acknowledged an orientation termed 'Reciprocator': 'I have come to recognise that the model (Facilitator–Regulator) is not linear but circular, with the intermediary group having a philosophy and identity of their own, as Reciprocators'. The Reciprocator is somewhat ambivalent about her pregnancy—although she is overjoyed about being pregnant, she has regrets about the changes a child will bring to her life. Although a deeper knowledge and understanding of the intricacies surrounding Raphael-Leff's model can only be acheived by further study of psychoanalytic theory, it presents an important dimension of psychological theory which is applicable to women in pregnancy and labour.

Raphael-Leff (1985) recognised the effects of 'increasing liberalisation of parental roles and child-care practices and conflicting pressures from … child-care experts and personal fulfilment advocates'. In addition, the views of professionals caring for women and their partners at this time may influence conscious and unconscious processes which affect individual perception and choice. Raphael-Leff (1991) has distinguished between Facilitators' and Regulators' perceptions of pain in labour. She suggests that for the Regulator, who incidentally may have planned her birth, pain is perceived as both a threat and a challenge. For the Regulator, maintenance of her self-esteem rests on her capacity to 'endure the torture stoically or (to make) a determined effort to deflect what she perceives as an inflicted agonising ordeal'. The indications for a Regulator experiencing internal satisfaction with the birth process if she has access to pharmacological methods of pain relief are apparent. The Facilitator, on the other hand, tries to control the pain herself, refusing pain relief as she is 'suffused with sensations she defines not as pain but as sensual excitement'. The Facilitator therefore finds benefit from non-pharmacological pain management such as 'support, reassurance, massage', as well as from adequate information-giving.

Raphael-Leff (1991) refers to what she terms the 'Introspection–Extraversion continuum', identifying how some women are preoccupied with the internal sensations experienced during labour, controlling pain by relaxation and breathing techniques, by 'going inside themselves'. On the other hand, some women 'seek external diversions', concentrating on the benefit gained via those supporting them in labour. The significance of the type of care provided in labour is demonstrated by the fact that the Regulator is shown to be dependent on human contact and the physical support of staff, whereas the 'introspective Facilitator' regards social contact as an intrusion and also resents verbal encouragement. The Facilitator–Regulator orientation could be seen as a typical personality dimension. However Raphael-Leff, perhaps naturally, resists any indication of the model being a theory of personality. She moreover suggests that orientations do in fact change with a subsequent baby, as changes in 'the inner world', emotional growth, resolution of inner conflicts and socio-economic factors influence the woman and her family, and additionally through changes which may be brought about by psychotherapy. On the other hand, many personality theories such as Eysenck's typology see individual characteristics as fixed components, and aspects of introversion or extraversion do not change. The possibility of change in individual characterisics relating to personality is an aspect which is frequently debated in the psychological arena.

Personality and pain perception

There is very little evidence available which specifically relates personality theory as presented by Eysenck and others—who suggest for example that personality differences are biologically based in the nervous system—to a woman's experience of pain in labour. The ability to compare and contrast such theories with that proposed by Raphael-Leff is therefore limited. One of the few studies undertaken some years ago, which set out to present an application of those measures which assess extraversion and introversion as applied to women in labour (Eysenck 1961), suggested that typically extroverts tolerate pain less well than introverts, the former 'giving voice' while the latter 'grin and bear it'.

It is perhaps interesting to note that Eysenck's study reflects the view of society at that time in that he compares married and unmarried mothers. The stigma of unmarried motherhood is evident, as the particular subject group were stated to be residents in 'three Moral Welfare Church of England homes'. The fact that society saw unmarried mothers as a group in need of 'moral welfare' may have had some influence on the perception of pain in labour by the individuals concerned. These young pregnant women may have had their suffering emphasised by the general negative attitudes towards them, inherent in society at the time. It was not uncommon for women of this era to have their baby adopted; their pain may thus have been accentuated by the loss of their infant. It is possible that a study involving a group such as this is recording their ability to 'grin and bear' their overall experience of pregnancy and childbirth, or alternatively their ability to 'give voice' to their feelings, and not solely recording their experience of pain during labour.

Wade et al (1992) showed that overall personality factors, as measured in terms of neuroticism and extraversion, did not influence the perception of pain sensation, particularly not in terms of pain intensity. However, certain personality traits were shown to influence the ways in which pain sufferers assessed the meaning of pain in their lives, and subsequently their levels of emotional suffering. In particular, assertiveness as a subfacet of extraversion was identified as important in predicting pain suffering. For example, highly assertive individuals demonstrated more obvious pain behaviour, and in addition received less response from family members when demonstrating such behaviour.

Personality is sometimes associated with pain perception as reflected in some areas of pain management. Latham (1988) reported on the use of certain personality assessment questionnaires in the treatment of patients within pain clinics. The Middlesex Hospital Questionnaire (Crown & Crispin 1966) is identified as a 'better measure of the personalities of pain patients' than many other personality inventories. This questionnaire 'highlights six different personality traits: free-floating anxiety, phobic anxiety, depression, hysteria, somatic complaints and obsessionality'. Personality questionnaires are used to develop a personality profile of patients attending pain clinics, which in some cases has been found to be helpful.

Assessing orientation?

There has been little suggestion as yet that personality profiling will be advantageous in assessing women for appropriate methods of pain relief in labour. Raphael-Leff (1983) and Sharp & Cooper (1992) each developed questionnaires which assessed the thoughts and feelings of women towards pregnancy, birth and the baby. These questionnaires have been used to identify Facilitator and Regulator orientations, as originally proposed by Raphael-Leff. The questionnaires are complex and lengthy and would be extremely cumbersome to use in midwifery practice. It is more appropriate to assess a woman's need for pain relief in labour through the use of an individual birth plan which has been discussed with a midwife whom she knows, and who in turn is aware of the psychological processes of childbirth.

There is some suggestion that Facilitators will be more satisfied with the labour experience if they use non-pharmacological methods of pain relief (Moore 1995, unpubl. data). This study demonstrated certain trends, indicating that Facilitators were less willing to use pethidine in labour, and less willing to accept the possible benefits when they did use it. Facilitators also appeared to be less willing to consider the use of epidural anaesthesia and were pleased when they did not use it. In addition, Facilitators

appeared to be more satisfied with the labour experience when using breathing and relaxation rather than pharmacological methods of pain relief. Raphael-Leff's Facilitator–Regulator model is a comprehensive theory acknowledging many of the psychological factors relevant to women's experience during the childbearing process, and concurring with observations inherent in midwifery theory and practice. In line with much of the evidence presented so far, the model acknowledges and supports many psychological factors which influence a woman's experience of childbirth.

The theory is typically complex, and readily conforms to representing those individual characteristics which differentiate people, while at the same time acknowledging uniqueness. It recognises the repercussions of aspects relating to control and self-efficacy, as well as the influence imposed by those individuals supporting a woman in labour, whether it be professional support or social support by family members. In fact, Raphael-Leff (1985) proposes orientations of fathering labelled 'Participator' and 'Renouncer', which further recognise the interactions between women and their partners. The Facilitator–Regulator model also recognises the types of coping strategies for dealing with pain in labour which certain individuals may adopt, together with the forms of pharmacological pain relief which would be appropriate. In this way, the theory increases knowledge of the possible consequences of the childbearing experience, and provides a model for predicting possible psychological outcome, as well as being a tool for predicting potential pathology. The Facilitator–Regulator model is a psychological development that is significant to midwifery practice, particularly when it is applied to the perception and relief of pain in labour.

There is little doubt that a recognition of the unconscious 'orientation' of particular women throughout pregnancy and childbirth by midwives would serve to identify and meet the needs of individuals. The potential for negative stereotyping and discrimination against certain groups of women by professionals would then be reduced. If midwives understand that a woman's expectations and plans for care in childbirth are not just fashionable whims predicted by the latest glossy magazine, then the midwifery profession can truly say that it is 'woman-centred'. Maternal orientations may therefore act as predictors for the provision of care in childbirth and, more specifically, for the management of pain relief in labour.

SUMMARY

The overall aim of *Changing Childbirth* (Department of Health 1993) is to bring about change in the provision of care in the maternity services, reinforcing the need for women to have choice and control over the type of care they receive. It is the case, however, that many women do not find it easy to make a real choice. One possible contributory factor is that women cannot readily appreciate their own unconscious needs. Although there is no suggestion that midwives need to become psychoanalysts, by understanding and acknowledging the significance of psychological processes it is anticipated that methods of pain relief appropriate to all women may be more readily assessed on an individual basis.

The influence of many elements of midwifery practice on the individual's experience of childbirth must also be recognised, as well as the significance of aspects of care such as quality of interaction and effective communication.

Good basic psychological care involves respect, compassion, reassurance, the giving of information, the provision of choice, the acknowledgement of concerns, the sharing of joys and sorrows. These are the components of good midwifery care … which (has) been embodied in concepts such as holistic care or empowering the parturient

(Niven 1992).

REFERENCES

Allport GW 1937 Personality: a psychological interpretation. Rinehart and Winston, New York

Allport G W 1961 Pattern and growth in personality. In: Gross R D 1993 Psychology: the science of mind and behaviour. Hodder and Stoughton, London

Baker A, Kenner A N 1993 Communication of pain: vocalisation as an indicator of the stage of labour. Australian and New Zealand Journal of Obstetrics and Gynaecology 33 (4): 384–385

Bibring G L 1959 Some considerations of the psychological processes of pregnancy. Psychoanalytic Study of the Child 14: 113–121

Bowlby J 1969 Attachment and loss: attachment, vol 1. Hogarth Press, London

British Medical Association and Royal Pharmaceutical Society 1994 British National Formulary 26. BMA/RPS, London

Cartwright A 1979 The dignity of labour. Tavistock, London

Chamberlain G, Wraight A, Steer P 1993 Pain and its relief in childbirth: the results of a national survey conducted by the National Birthday Trust. Churchill Livingstone, Edinburgh

Condon J T 1993 The assessment of antenatal emotional attachment: development of a questionnaire instrument. British Journal of Medical Psychology 66: 167–183

Combes G, Schonveld A 1992 Life will never be the same again: learning to be a first time parent. Health Education Authority, London

Craig K D 1994 Emotional aspects of pain. In: Wall P D, Melzack R (eds) Textbook of pain. Churchill Livingstone, Edinburgh

Department of Health 1993 Changing childbirth, Part 1. Report of the expert maternity group. HMSO, London

Dick Read G 1944 Childbirth without fear. Harper, New York

Donnison J 1988 Midwives and medical men: a history of the struggle for the control of childbirth. Historical Publications, London

Eysenck H 1953 The structure of human personality. Methuen, London

Eysenck S B G 1961 Personality and pain assessment in childbirth of married and unmarried mothers. Journal of Mental Science 123: 417–429

Green J M, Kitzinger V J, Coupland V A 1990 Stereotypes of childbearing women: a look at some evidence. Midwifery 6: 125–132

Inch S 1982 Birthrights: a parents' guide to modern childbirth. Hutchinson, London

Keefe F J, Wilkins R H, Cook W A, Crisson J E, Muhlbaier L H 1986 Depression, pain and pain behaviour. Journal of Consulting and Clinical Psychology 54: 665–669

Keirse M, Enkin M, Lumley J 1989 Social and professional support during childbirth. In: Chalmers I, Enkin M, Keirse M J N C (eds) Effective care in pregnancy and childbirth, vol 1. Oxford University Press, Oxford, p 805–814

Kimmel D C 1980 Adulthood and ageing. In: Niven N (ed) Health psychology. Churchill Livingstone, Edinburgh

Kirkham M 1989 Midwives and information giving during labour. In: Robinson S, Thomson A (eds) Midwives, research and childbirth, vol 1. Chapman and Hall, London, p 117–138

Kitzinger S 1991 The midwife challenge. Pandora, London

Lamaze F 1970 Painless childbirth, psychoprophylaxis method. Regnery, Chicago

Latham J 1988 Pain control. Austen Cornish, London

Lewis T L T, Chamberlain G V P (eds) 1990 Obstetrics by ten teachers. Edward Arnold, London

MacArthur C, Lewis M, Knox E G, Crawford E S 1990 Epidural anaesthesia and long-term backache after childbirth. British Medical Journal 309: 9–12

Mackey M C, Stepans M E F 1994 Women's evaluations of their labour and delivery nurses. Journal of Obstetrics, Gynaecological and Neonatal Nursing 23 (5): 413–420

Macmillan M 1995 Men at birth, a survey conducted by the Royal College of Midwives. RCM, London

Melzack R, Taenzer P, Feldman P, Kinch R A 1981 Labour is still painful after prepared childbirth training. Canadian Medical Association Journal 125: 357–363

Melzack R, Wall P 1988 The challenge of pain. Penguin Books, London

Moir 1986 Pain relief in labour. Churchill Livingstone, Edinburgh

Mountcastle V B 1980 Medical physiology. Mosby, St Louis

Niven C 1985 How helpful is the presence of the husband at childbirth. Journal of Reproductive and Infant Psychology 3: 45–53

Niven C 1988 Labour pain: long term recall and consequences. Journal of Reproductive and Infant Psychology 6: 83–87

Niven C 1992 Psychological care for families: before during and after birth. Butterworth-Heinemann, Oxford

Niven C 1994 Coping with labour pain: the midwife's role. Chapman and Hall, London

O'Driscoll K, Meagher D 1980 Active management of labour. Bailliere Tindall, London

O'Driscoll M 1994 Midwives, childbirth and sexuality; men and sex. British Journal of Midwifery 2 (2): 74–76

Page L 1988 The midwife's role in modern health care. In: Kitzinger S (ed) The midwife challenge. Pandora Press, London

Phares E J 1976 Locus of control in personality. General Learning Fairway Press, Morristown, NJ

Quine L, Rutter D R, Gowen S 1993 Women's satisfaction with the birth experience: a prospective study of social and psychological predictors. Journal of Reproductive and Infant Psychology 11: 107–113

Rajan L 1993 Perceptions of pain and pain relief in labour: the gulf between experience and observation. Midwifery 9: 136–145

Raphael-Leff J 1983 Facilitators and regulators: two approaches to mothering. British Journal of Medical Psychology 56: 376–390

Raphael-Leff J 1985 Facilitators and regulators; participators and renouncers: mothers' and fathers' orientations towards pregnancy and parenthood. Journal of Psychosomatic Obstetrics and Gynaecology 4: 169–184

Raphael-Leff J 1991 Psychological processes of childbearing. Chapman and Hall, London

Raphael-Leff J 1993 Pregnancy the inside story. Sheldon Press, London

Reading A E, Cox D N 1985 Psychological predictors of labour pain. Pain 22: 309–315

Robertson A 1994 Empowering women: teaching active birth in the 90's. Ace Graphics, Sevenoaks

Robson K, Kumar R 1980 Delayed onset of maternal affection after childbirth. British Journal of Psychiatry 136: 347–353

Rotter J 1966 Generalised expectancies for internal versus external control of reinforcement. Psychological Monographs, 80, 1 (609): 1–28

Scott-Palmer J, Skevington S M 1981 Pain during childbirth and menstruation: a study of locus of control. Journal of Psychosomatic Research 25 (3): 151–155

Sharp H M, Cooper S A 1992 Ideal expectations versus outcome characteristics within a representative population of primiparous women. Paper presented at the 6th International Conference of the Marce Society, Edinburgh, 2–4 Sept.

Skevington S M, Wilkes P 1992 Choice and control: a comparative study of childbirth preparation classes. Journal of Reproductive and Infant Psychology 10: 19–28

Turk D C, Wack J T, Kerns R D 1985 An empirical examination of the pain behaviour construct. Journal of Behavioural Medicine 8: 119–130

Ussher J M 1993 The psychology of the female body. Routledge, London and New York

Wade J B, Dougherty L M, Hart R P, Rajii A, Price D D 1992 A canonical correlation analysis of the influence of neuroticism and extraversion on chronic pain, suffering and pain behaviour. Pain 51: 67–73

Weisenberg M 1994 Cognitive aspects of pain. In: Wall P D, Melzack R (eds) Textbook of pain. Churchill Livingstone, Edinburgh

5

Management of labour pain by midwives: a historical perspective

Thelma Bamfield

LEARNING OUTCOMES

At the end of this chapter the reader will have

- **considered some of the historical features of the management of pain in labour by midwives**

- **considered the background to differing perspectives of the management of labour pain**

- **identified methods of pain relief used in the past and the rationale for their use at the time**

- **an increased awareness of the influences of traditional views of pain management on current management of pain in labour**

- **considered the influence of medicalisation of childbirth on pain experience in labour**

- **an introduction to the relationship between 'natural childbirth', relief of anxiety and effective support to pain relief in labour.**

There is an inverse ratio between the need for analgesia and the quality of care in a delivery unit

(O'Driscoll 1975).

This chapter offers one perspective of the history of attempts by midwives to help women cope with the sensations experienced during normal labour. The focus is on the years following World War II when births in hospital were increasing due to lack of domestic help and suitable home accommodation, and before the dramatic increase in medical intervention in the 1960s and 1970s, when women undergoing induction and augmentation of labour became 'distraught with pain' (Myles 1975). Material is drawn from an ongoing study of women's childbearing experiences in a local and national context. Archive material from some of Birmingham's maternity hospitals, though incomplete, demonstrates clear trends in the use of drugs for sedation and pain relief. Over the same period of time there was, paradoxically, increased recognition of, and attention to, the psychological dimensions of pain perception.

THE BACKGROUND: ANAESTHESIA AND ANALGESIA FOR BIRTH

Early efforts to relieve pain, notably James Young Simpson's experiments with ether and chloroform in 1847, focused on the moment of birth. The main reason for this is that the doctor who would administer the drugs was unlikely to have been present for the whole of the labour:

Don't panic about sending for the doctor. Nurse knows exactly when it will be necessary. Trust her and be as calm and as brave as you can. And then, at last, just as you are wondering how long it is going on and whether you really can bear it, the doctor is there, and there is a whiff of chloroform for you, and when you wake up, Baby has come and is waiting for you to take him in your arms

(Allied Newspapers Ltd, undated, c. 1920).

Whether he was called in at exactly the right moment by a maternity nurse, or summoned in an emergency by a midwife, what Beinart (1990) refers to as 'the pioneering spirit of the early chloroformists' may have been inspired to some extent by the doctor's need to be perceived as a hero, coming to a woman's aid at her most desperate hour—'humanity, with its noblest gesture has stepped in to slay the dragon and so free the princess' (Read 1943).

Chloroform administered 'à la reine' aimed to maintain the woman's active cooperation with pushing, but to make her unconscious for the actual birth: '… towards the end of the 2nd stage of labour, and when the head is crowned, the patient is completely anaesthetised for a short time, but otherwise the aim is merely to render her muzzy' (Clyne 1963). Obstetricians presumed that labour was most painful when its processes

were visible to an observer. 'The pain is most severe during the actual birth of the child, because there is then both the strongest contraction and most marked retraction of the uterus as well as the greatest distension of the soft parts' (Fairbairn 1918).

It is not clear whether this perception was shared by the women, but the quest for an analgesic which could be administered by midwives still focused on the second stage. The trial set up by the British (later Royal) College of Obstetricians and Gynaecologists (BCOG) investigated chiefly chloroform and nitrous oxide ('gas') and air. Although Minnitt's apparatus, which was ultimately approved, was designed for use throughout labour (British Medical Journal 1934), the BCOG's ruling that two qualified persons must be present when it was in use (one to administer the gas while the other maintained a sterile field for the delivery) effectively meant that its use was largely restricted to late second stage, and to hospital practice. The equipment was also heavy, bulky and expensive, further hindering its uptake by district midwives.

Some midwives were reported as being 'prejudiced against gas and air, holding that it prolongs labour, makes the patient more difficult to control, or simply that it is unnecessary' (Ministry of Health 1949). A later textbook suggests that such reservations may not have been without foundation: '… as the head begins to crown and to distend the vulva, the patient [using gas and air] may become unmanageable and it requires considerable tact and self-control on the part of the midwife to control the patient at times' (Brown et al 1962).

Gas and air contained only half as much oxygen as atmospheric air. Trichloroethylene (Trilene) vapour in air in concentrations of 0.5% or 0.35% left oxygen intake virtually unchanged, and so was considered much safer if maternal oxygen-carrying capacity or placental perfusion were compromised (Da Cruz 1967). Tecota Mark 6 and Emotril inhalers were approved by the Central Midwives' Board (CMB) in 1955, but Trilene does not seem to have been popular. Less than 1% of women used it in one hospital in 1959, while 72% received gas and air (Lordswood Maternity

Hospital (LMH) birth registers). Nitrous oxide with oxygen was used for situations such as premature labour, breech deliveries and fetal distress, but could not be administered by midwives on their own responsibility until the Entonox apparatus was approved by the CMB in 1966. Use of gas and air immediately declined.

The first survey of women's experiences of maternity care took up the issue of pain relief. The Joint Committee of the Royal College of Obstetricians and Gynaecologists and the Population Investigation Committee (1948; hereafter Joint Committee) examined the services available to, and utilised by, all women delivering in 1 week in 1946. They found that 'of the large towns, Birmingham [was] most successful, securing analgesia in 71% of hospital confinements'. This compared favourably with, for example, London's 48%. Included in this calculation were gas and air, chloroform, Trilene, twilight sleep (morphine with scopolamine, an amnesic), and spinal and general anaesthetics. Classing all these interventions as 'successful' implies that for a woman to be rendered unconscious or even muzzy for the birth of her child was the ultimate aim. Perhaps there is again an element of observer perspective.

Part of the committee's remit had been to examine reasons for the falling birth rate in a country trying to re-establish itself and its empire after World War II. Its conclusion that one reason was 'unnecessary pain during labour' may have been rather naive, and the recommendation that one way of overcoming this would be the provision of more gas and air machines appears to arise more from members' preconceived ideas than from anything said by the women who were interviewed.

The questions which elicited the information on which these conclusions are supposedly based reflect the underlying medical assumption not only that pain is an inevitable component of labour but also that the way to alleviate it is with medication. Women were not actually asked whether they wanted drugs, and the question about whether they thought that 'anything more could have been done to make your delivery or confinement more satisfactory' is placed directly

after the one asking what they were given 'to relieve the pain' (Joint Committee 1948). Such leading questions make it unsound to draw any firm conclusions about the representativeness of those who were not given analgesia and complained that 'no attempt had been made to relieve their labour pains', still less what kind of intervention they thought might have been beneficial to them.

'ALLEVIATING ANXIETY': SEDATION AND ANALGESIA IN LABOUR

Morphine and scopolamine were the only drugs identified in the Joint Committee survey which would be used in the first stage, when medication was sometimes necessary if labour was not progressing normally. Before operative intervention was a safe option, and when methods of inducing or accelerating labour were unreliable, great faith was placed in the restorative powers of food and sleep. Opium in its various forms was considered the best treatment in emergency situations such as haemorrhage and eclampsia, as well as for uterine inertia and 'dry labour', when prolonged rupture of the membranes was thought to cause exceptional distress.

Sedatives also had a long history of use when progress was slow, and could be given by midwives on their own responsibility. Drugs such as chloral hydrate and potassium or sodium bromide, used either alone or frequently in combination, were considered valuable 'to induce sleep, dull the pains, and relax rigidity of the soft parts' (Fairbairn 1918). The Sorrento Maternity Hospital (SMH) birth registers suggest a dramatic escalation in the use of sedatives towards the end of 1945. First recorded in July of that year, with indications such as 'antepartum haemorrhage' or 'delay in labour' they were soon given to increasing numbers of women in normal labour. The next years with complete sets of registers show that 73% of women received sedatives in 1948, and 82% in 1949.

Margaret Myles (1956) recommended sedatives as 'being particularly useful for the excitable or apprehensive woman at the beginning of labour'. Whether this indication explains their increased use raises further questions, particularly as Myles goes on to warn that 'neither [chloral hydrate nor potassium bromide] has any analgesic action nor will they *induce sleep* if the woman has frequent painful contractions' (italics added). It would seem that there was either a dramatic escalation in the proportion of excitable or nervous women, or a change in emphasis of care during labour, with an expectation that women should sleep through it.

The analgesia which sedatives did not offer was to be provided by pethidine, the optimum dosages of which, like the preferred drugs themselves, were evidently arrived at by trial and error. In 1944 women were being given initial doses of 200 mg, followed by second doses of 50 or 100 mg after an hour or two; one received 200 mg 50 minutes before delivery, with no ill effects recorded (SMH birth registers). Once midwives were permitted to administer the drug on their own responsibility, a total of 200 mg could be given to any one woman, with an initial dose usually not exceeding 100 mg. Subsequent hospital practice reverted to the earlier regime: 'Pethidine, 100 mg, is not considered to be adequate, as an initial dose, by many labour ward sisters: 150 to 200 mg has a deeper and more lasting effect: repeat doses of 100 mg are given every two, three or four hours, depending on the needs of the patient' (Myles 1968). In one hospital opiates were given freely, either instead of or in addition to pethidine: 78% received one or other or both in 1955, 81% in 1957 (Queen Elizabeth Hospital (QEH) birth registers). It would seem that the aim was to keep women in labour in a state of stupefaction.

The use of sedatives declined as pethidine was used more often. Initial claims for pethidine that, in addition to relieving pain, it 'induces sleep, and by its antispasmodic action relaxes plain muscle, including that of the lower uterine segment; it therefore facilitates dilatation of the os' (Myles 1956, 1961), were later modified (Myles 1968). Whatever its precise mode of action, and despite the rebukes of anaesthetists (Crawford 1984) regarding correct terminology, midwives continued to refer to pethidine as 'sedation'. As far as they were concerned, any influence on progress of labour or in relief of pain was less important than its soporific effects; above all it was a more effective sedative. Even in 1994, midwives were reported as saying that one of their principle reasons for administering pethidine early in labour was 'to alleviate anxiety' (Niven 1994).

Only inhalational analgesia was actually regarded by midwives specifically as pain relief. Women who declined to use it were recorded as having refused analgesia, even if they had received pethidine (LMH birth registers), and if inhalational analgesia was not administered, an explanation was included. Even women who delivered 5 minutes after admission are recorded as having received gas and air. It is clear that women expected, or were expected, to be offered pharmaceutical pain relief in labour. Drugs and methods of administration may have become more sophisticated, but arguably no less experimental, since 1959, but the same expectation is implicit in maternity service provision today.

The report of the Working Party on Midwives had claimed that: 'A very large and increasing proportion of women today wish to have labour rendered as painless as possible and public opinion is on their side' (Ministry of Health 1949). If drug administration is the measure of success, women's wishes were fulfilled. Within the next 10 years, less than 6% of women at one hospital gave birth without any form of medication, and half of those had precipitate labours, or were admitted in the second stage or with the child already born (LMH birth registers).

'NATURAL CHILDBIRTH' AND THE WORK OF GRANTLY DICK READ

Some of the women reported by the Joint Committee to have refused analgesia stated that they had been trained in the methods advocated by Grantly Dick Read. Read's embryonic thoughts about 'natural childbirth' were formulated in 1919, and refined through extensive clinical experience before his first book was published in 1932 (Read 1959). By 1935 his ideas had gained sufficient acceptance for him to contribute a chapter on 'The influence of the emotions upon pregnancy and parturition' to a standard medical textbook (Browne 1944). It is impossible to know how widespread use of his methods was. Jenny Kitzinger (1990) has documented how the Natural Childbirth Association (NCA), formed in 1956 to promote his ideas, had within a few years espoused a different approach to preparation for birth and adopted a less radical title—the National Childbirth Trust (NCT). Read's methods, however, formed the basis for the 'relaxation classes' offered by hospitals and welfare centres from the 1940s up to the present day.

Read's basic premise was that ignorance of bodily functions and the process of labour leads to fear when contractions are first experienced. Fear results in tension, tension results in pain, the experience of pain leads to fear of the next contraction, and the cycle is repeated. Removing ignorance was the key to removing fear, and teaching relaxation techniques could break the cycle and alter perception of the sensations as painful.

The Working Party, which maintained that women wanted drugs to render labour as painless as possible, at the same time noted 'that the great majority of young women of all classes are deplorably ignorant of the functioning of the sexual organs and that the mists of tabu and superstition … cling … tenaciously to this subject' (Ministry of Health 1949). They were actually referring to student nurses, who might, however 'ignorant and possibly prudishly brought-up', be assumed to be somewhat less ill-informed about bodily functions than the general population of women of childbearing age, but the significance of this evidently escaped the Working Party. Early editions of Read's book had emphasised the ignorance of young women at the time: '… their bodies are a mystery and labour an incomprehensible activity too difficult to discuss' (Read 1943). This section does not appear in later editions (Read 1959). It was noted in 1961 that women were far better informed than in previous years about their bodies (Central Health Services Council Standing Maternity and Midwifery Advisory Committee 1961; hereafter Central Health Services Council). Nevertheless, childbirth was still considered to be 'private, undignified, and disgusting' by many in the 1950s and

1960s (Kitzinger 1990). Change in attitudes and awareness was gradual, and there can be no doubt that fear grounded in ignorance of the processes of labour was a major factor in the experiences of women giving birth in the 1940s.

In the 1980s and 1990s it would seem impossible to remain ignorant about sex and childbirth. Women can be expected to have at least a basic understanding, and antenatal classes explain the physiology of labour, and yet there is still evidence of the reality of the 'fear–tension–pain' syndrome. A recent report (Green 1993) of a large prospective study concluded that findings concerning anxiety 'unambiguously' supported Grantly Dick Read's position: 'Anxiety about the pain of labour was a strong predictor of negative experiences during labour, lack of satisfaction with the birth, and poor emotional well-being postnatally'. Women tended to experience what they expected to, whether that was a lot of pain or a little.

Read's concern to enable women to approach childbirth with confidence appears to make sense today, and he was ahead of his time in many other ways as well. He advocated breast feeding on demand, and rooming-in, if mothers wanted it, at a time when babies were kept in nurseries and only brought out at regular intervals; feeding rigidly by the clock was the norm. Most importantly, he drew attention to psychological and emotional aspects of labour and birth as well as pregnancy and the postnatal period, and advocated the husband's company during labour as long as he had been 'interested with [his wife] in the preparation for labour' (Read 1950), a practice that was not widespread until the 1980s. His belief that women needed to be awake and aware as they gave birth arose in the context of chloroform being given for delivery, but has relevance to the more recent debate about the virtues of epidural rather than general anaesthesia for Caesarean section. His comment about spinal anaesthesia—'an offspring is produced by a magician from a paralyzed birth canal' (Read 1959)—suggests a feeling of deprivation similar to that subsequently expressed by some women who had epidurals (Crawford 1972, Billewicz-Driemel & Milne 1976).

So many of Read's ideas are now accepted that it is important to consider why his most fundamental belief—that women could, and deserved to, achieve fulfilment and satisfaction in giving birth to their babies—has been ignored or even ridiculed. Why was his 'a lone voice crying in the wilderness' (Read 1943)?

One problem is that his writings are set in an intensely religious context. Bringing forth a new life may have another dimension than the purely physical one, but spiritual aspects of birth evoke an uncomfortable response in an age which values the rational and the scientific. Metaphysical ideas are incongruous in a hospital, and anyone considering them important would be unlikely to articulate them in such a setting.

Read has been criticised as 'working within a simplistic, pseudo-evolutionary opposition of nature and culture, primitive and civilised' (Cosslett 1994). He emphasised that motherhood was the 'realisation of [women's] highest ambition, the fulfilment of their instinctive urge and the ultimate perfection of their bodily functions' (Read 1943), and reconciled this neatly with the prevailing ideology of woman as homemaker: 'Pregnancy should be as normal for a woman as wage earning is for a man'. Birth was not 'naturally' painful, and culturally induced fears could be overcome by training during pregnancy and support during labour. There is still, yet again, an element of the (male) observer's perspective, rather than that of the woman herself.

Ideological concerns apart, it may simply be, of course, that the method itself was unable to deliver what it promised. The recommended preparation consisted of exercises to encourage suppleness, good posture and general physical fitness, relaxation and controlled deep breathing (Read 1950). The physiotherapists who developed the approach evidently found the rather vague instructions unsatisfactory, and taught a more structured method of relaxation, contracting and relaxing groups of muscles in turn, and three levels of breathing for uterine contractions of progressive strength (Heardman 1958).

The fact that the NCT, founded to promote Read's teachings, abandoned them in favour of a more active approach (Kitzinger 1990) suggests that even motivated women found them inadequate, for whatever reason, to enable them to achieve 'natural childbirth'. The Lamaze method ('psychoprophylaxis') which they adopted maintained that the standard approach to relaxation actually increased sensitivity to pain (Karmel 1965). Psychoprophylaxis needs intensive training and rehearsal, and is likely therefore to appeal to an even smaller number of committed women.

'Relaxation classes' were, nevertheless, to become an accepted part of antenatal care. A textbook for midwives advocated the teaching of progressive relaxation during pregnancy: 'The woman who can relax has a shorter and easier first stage, and in the second stage her pelvic floor will offer less resistance' (Johnstone 1946). Clearly, tangible benefits were perceived for both mothers and midwives.

One of the Birmingham hospitals introduced relaxation classes in 1944 (Birmingham Maternity Hospital (BMH) annual report), but their wider availability depended on the commitment of those who were experienced in the methods and prepared to pass on their expertise to the midwives who would have to teach them. Another hospital began programmes for expectant mothers in 1947, and the physiotherapist gave her services voluntarily. With the inception of the NHS the following year she was officially appointed to the staff, and classes were transferred from the antenatal clinic to a local church hall to accommodate the increasing numbers. Visitors from all over the country and abroad came to observe (LMH medical officer's report July 1968), and she published a slim volume explaining the method (Madders 1958).

'REASSURING THE NERVOUS PATIENTS': MOTHERCRAFT AND RELAXATION CLASSES

The principle of relaxation for labour was evidently becoming widely accepted at the same time as the use of medication was increasing so dramatically. There seems to be no simple explanation for this, but a number of contributory factors can be identified.

Not all women had access to classes. The Maternity Services Committee deplored the fact that 'hospitals and general practitioners seldom arranged for their patients to receive health education or ante-natal exercises unless they themselves provided special classes' (Ministry of Health 1959). The women would not necessarily have attended if they had been available, but the fragmented provision of antenatal care made uptake problematic.

An early edition of one textbook takes it for granted that professionals will build up a relationship with the prospective mother during pregnancy. This was important in order to establish 'that complete confidence in her doctor and midwife which is of the greatest importance to the patient, and without which her willing co-operation cannot be secured' (Johnstone 1946). A later edition (Johnstone 1962) goes on, somewhat plaintively: 'It may be added that the building of confidence is best achieved when the patient is under continuous care by the same doctor and the same midwife throughout pregnancy, labour and the puerperium. This ideal may be hard to obtain in a modern urban society, but it should certainly be aimed at.'

The ideal of continuity is thus perceived as the best way of increasing a woman's confidence, but in her attendants, rather than herself. Another textbook emphasised that *every effort should be made to reassure the patient and to gain her confidence and co-operation* (Browne 1944; emphasis in original).

By 1953, lack of suitable accommodation was resulting in 'a very long waiting list of patients wishing to take advantage of the relaxation classes for preparation for childbirth' (LMH statistics, April 1953). The situation was eased in June of that year when all the welfare centres in the city started to hold their own classes, and some of the women on the waiting list were diverted elsewhere.

This is not always in agreement with the wishes of the patient, who often prefers to attend our relaxation class. This enables her to become acquainted with the hospital staff and also with the mothers she is likely to meet during her confinement in hospital. In our experience this plays an important part in reassuring the nervous patients in their mental attitude towards the expected confinement in hospital

(LMH medical officer's report, July 1953).

Antenatal classes not only offer reassurance, but also serve the purpose of ensuring compliance with antenatal supervision and hospital regimes; they offer 'an unrivalled opportunity for putting across obstetric propaganda from authoritative sources' to an unquestioning target audience (Tew 1995). According to Browne (1944), it was necessary to explain why the administration of hypnotic and analgesic drugs in labour had to be limited: 'Every woman could in theory be given a painless labour, but there would be very few live babies'. One of the advantages of teaching a woman relaxation during pregnancy was so that she would be able to 'co-operate at the time of her labour and get the maximum value out of her efforts' (Johnstone 1946). There is nothing intrinsically problematic about the notion of a woman cooperating with the professionals looking after her, of course: a frightened woman wastes valuable energy, and the calm, controlled delivery of the baby's head and shoulders benefits both mother and child. It is only when the content of the 'relaxation' classes themselves is examined that there is cause for concern.

The Maternity Services Committee felt that 'clinical methods' such as 'natural childbirth' or relaxation were 'outside [their] terms of reference', and that they 'would not wish to express an opinion' on their value, but endorsed the generally held view that 'health education and mothercraft instruction should be available to all expectant mothers' (Ministry of Health 1959). This recommendation must be seen in the context of the traditional perception of antenatal education, which targeted pregnant women in order to ensure the health of the next generation: 'The mother is the executive in the nurture of her family, and concentration on her is a corollary to the wide objective of all the services engaged in supervising the rising generation. On her health, efficiency and knowledge of elementary hygiene depends the health of her family' (Fairbairn 1944).

The focus of 'mothercraft classes' remained on acceptable standards of diet, hygiene and baby care, and bringing 'expectant mothers ... into contact with the other health services' (Joint Committee 1948). This report recommended that inhalational analgesia should be offered to every woman fit to receive it, and that instruction in its use should be included in antenatal education. They did not mention relaxation, and neither did the Working Party on Midwives report (Ministry of Health 1949), which implicitly endorsed the Joint Committee's view. They expressed concern that in 1946 only one in five practising midwives was trained to give gas and air, which they believed to be effective as long as the woman had been prepared antenatally. By the time the Maternity Services Committee reported (Ministry of Health 1959), although relaxation classes were well established, the 'good maternity service' which they outline does not include them, but only includes demonstrations of analgesic apparatus during mothercraft sessions.

Probably the best clue available to the content of actual classes is from *Myles' Textbooks for Midwives*, which are of value because they include 'the talk (or the demonstration) as given'. The books were standard texts for many years and it is likely that sessions similar to the ones suggested were widespread. The talk on 'what happens during labour?' includes reassurance that sedatives will be given as soon as they are really needed. The relaxation demonstration incorporates good posture and pelvic exercises, and then, with the women lying on their backs, suggests: 'Close your eyes gently (don't screw them up tightly) and imagine you are lying under a tree on a lawn on a warm summer day. The leaves are rustling in the breeze, which brings the scent of honeysuckle; the sun is warm, and you feel tired and drowsy. Allow your lower jaw to drop …' (Myles 1956); and so on until the women fall asleep.

The next session is the 'rehearsal of use of analgesia machines': 'We start off by getting you to relax, and then when (sic) you need some relief, we will give you a sedative which will probably make you sleep. Later on you will, if you require it be given a second dose of the sedative, and when the effect of it is wearing off, the midwife will give you gas' (Myles 1956).

The pleasant nature of the gas and the sensations it gives are repeatedly emphasised; indeed, one of the purposes of the rehearsal is 'to arouse

enthusiasm for the analgesic' (Myles 1956). It is significant that, although the content of the 'talks as given' was modified considerably over the years, in response to the interest in psychoprophylaxis by (lay) NCT teachers (Myles 1968), and later to the active management of labour (Myles 1975), this particular purpose remained unchanged. To some extent the mode of administration is the reason for the need to arouse enthusiasm for the analgesic itself, but there is nothing in these talks to give women any confidence in their ability to labour and give birth undrugged. Indeed the underlying message is that relaxation will make the drugs more effective, rather than the other way around.

Read himself admitted that many women find that a relaxed state cannot be maintained when contractions intensify. He identified two particular phases, corresponding with the onset of the active and transition stages, when there is danger that a woman who has been in control may be overwhelmed by the sensations. In this event, he suggested that administration of a sedative or pethidine, or an inhalational analgesic, could help to numb the senses and relieve pain-causing tensions (Read 1950).

It is undoubtedly true that many women have achieved satisfying birth experiences after receiving such drugs, but equally true that many have found them unpleasant and counter-productive; the side-effects of pethidine, for example, are 'nausea, vomiting, disorientation and mental confusion' (O'Driscoll 1975). The surf-riding analogy may be a useful one: remaining on top of contractions is like riding a wave, a sensation of being borne along by immense forces, and requires calm alertness and intense concentration. 'If you panic—you will be submerged' (Karmel 1965). This loss of control is more likely to happen if analgesics have been given. Sheila Kitzinger (1967) makes a similar point, and compares having a baby in a doped condition to driving a car while semiconscious or under the influence of powerful drugs. Although well-intentioned, the administration of sedatives to help a woman 'go on controlling her own relaxation' (Heardman 1973) could have the opposite effect. 'When a woman is dozey from sedation, it is far harder for her to stay in touch with her labour. It is much more likely that she will willingly hand herself over to others' (Brook 1976).

The acceptance of medication, the implied passivity of the labouring woman, even the fact that the required state of relaxation was best achieved in bed, may mean that from the outset Read's methods were bound to fail. There may also have been an unanticipated side-effect: an increase in back problems as a result of taking to bed earlier in labour (Myles 1968). The fervent belief that '95 per cent of women should give birth to their children without danger or discomfort to themselves or injury to the baby' (Read 1950), may simply have been deluded, or fraudulent. But it is worth considering some of the other factors influencing its potential success or failure.

FEAR, TENSION AND PAIN: LABOUR AND BIRTH IN HOSPITAL

Read himself (1959) pointed out that 'however well prepared and confident in her ability to achieve a satisfactory and natural birth a woman may be, ultimately her success depends on each individual of the team of people to whose influence she has been subjected during the changing phases of her reproductive activity'. Indeed any pregnant woman's confidence may easily be undermined, and the risks are increased the more professionals she comes in contact with. The new National Health Service endorsed the existing fragmented provision of maternity care, which ensured that many women delivering in hospital would never have met their attendants before.

One of the complaints made about midwives was that women who were taught relaxation antenatally were not able/enabled to use it during labour because 'the labour ward staff do not believe in it' (Central Health Services Council 1961). Some physiotherapists tried to attend to help put the theory into practice (BMH annual report 1946, Heardman 1958, 1973), but presumably the effects of such a policy would be marginal to the experience of the majority of women. A survey carried out for the Maternity Services Committee had reported that 'if expectations are created which are not fulfilled, bitter disappointment will be felt, and resentment or even panic may ensue during labour' (Central Council for Health Education 1957). No answers were offered to this particular problem.

She expects to practise what she has been taught and has rehearsed during pregnancy, eg relaxation and controlled breathing, and should be encouraged to do so. Some women feel very deeply regarding being permitted (sic) to experience what is commonly known as 'natural childbirth' with the profound joy in hearing their baby's first cry. Although the midwife may think it is more humane to administer inhalational analgesia she must respect and comply with the mother's wishes which, *in this instance*, will have no untoward effect on mother or child

(Myles 1961; italics added).

(This passage appears unchanged in 1968 and 1975, but the first sentence is omitted from the latter edition.) A report based on accounts of birth from nearly 5000 women, over a period of 25 years, commented: 'Too often women are pressured or even forced to take sleeping drugs against their will' (Close 1980). Close also noted that 'the idea that all patients (including women in labour) *must* sleep at night is still very prevalent' among some members of hospital staff, and indeed a midwifery textbook stated that: 'If labour begins in the evening she should be settled in bed with a sedative' (Da Cruz 1967). 'Humane', perhaps, but it is not clear who was expected to benefit from such a policy. Once again, it would appear that the perceptions of attendants sometimes dictated management, rather than the woman's needs.

This paternalistic approach permeates the literature, always implicit but sometimes more overt. Another textbook, written by obstetricians, discusses the difficulties of protecting patients from 'the advice and attentions of kindly but ignorant relatives':

… many of these views on midwifery have been handed down from generation to generation and are firmly fixed in the patient's mind, almost as superstitions, so that the midwife will achieve nothing by merely dismissing these views and stating her own. She must attempt to show that she is interested in them but she must explain the reason why her own view is better

(Brown et al 1962).

Perhaps the medical profession was seeking to use midwives to extend their influence over women's lives, but in labour it could be a power struggle between women and the midwives themselves. Some of the women's 'views on midwifery' related to the use of drugs. Mrs JC, aged 71, recalls refusing gas and air for her fifth confinement:

'I said I'm not having that, and she, that's when she gave me a swipe, "You'll do as you're told," she said. She gave me a swipe across the backside. But I didn't have it. I brought 'em all natural, just as I wanted to.'

Mrs JC's eyes gleam with triumph as she tells her story. Her victory was possible perhaps because she was in her own home; women in hospital may not have been so fortunate.

Even in the 1990s, women are reported as being willing to put themselves into the hands of the professionals who 'know best' (Bluff & Holloway 1994). Their mothers and grandmothers were even less likely to question expert power, and before the women's movement were even more effectively socialised into feminine compliance and passivity. Handbooks stressed the importance of obeying orders: the exercises 'should *never* be attempted without the consent of the doctor' (Heardman 1958). Even Kathleen Vaughan (1951), a vociferous proponent of active birth, with squatting or kneeling positions for delivery, emphasised: 'Remember you *must* co-operate with your doctor and nurse. Do just as they wish.' (Emphases in originals.) She neglected to discuss what a woman should do in the face of opposition from her attendants.

Midwives clearly did develop strategies, short of outright assault, for dealing with women reluctant to submit to the hospital regime. Myles (1968) made the point that some women trained in psychoprophylaxis 'have been encouraged to believe that they are in control during labour and may refuse sedatives or advice'. Such women needed to be 'handled' with 'the utmost tact … *These women* do not expect to be left alone at any time and much of the alleged success of psychoprophylaxis stems from the constant supervision and professional companionship they receive from midwives during labour' (emphasis added). Such barely concealed hostility makes it clear that any woman imagining that she could beat the system by having one-to-one attention from a midwife, rather than being sedated and left alone, was likely to be given a hard time.

Outright opposition is not the only way to sabotage successful use of relaxation; lack of support is quite enough. Copstick et al (1985, 1986) found that most women used the techniques they had been taught at the beginning of labour, but without support and encouragement were unable to continue as labour progressed. A woman who has prepared herself for childbirth deserves 'suitable attendance when she needs it—to exhort her to further effort and to encourage her or to correct any faults that occur' (Heardman 1958). While for a few this support may simply take the form of acknowledgement and praise, for many it will include reinforcement and reiteration as contractions intensify. This means that the woman must not only not be left alone, but must have with her throughout labour someone who is committed to helping her achieve the birth experience she hoped for. We know that this was not the case in the period under review. Not only was supportive companionship lacking, but women were often left completely alone:

'Well, they just left me to get on with it in this nursing home, and it was quite shocking to me. I sort of had to, sort of think, er, what was happening to me. Put two and two together. I knew when the waters had broken, and just after, I knew she was being born, and instead of holding back, my mother had told me to press hard and get her into the world quickly, you know, which I did. And in doing that I caused myself to have to have some stitches. Whereas if I'd have been told to hold back a bit perhaps I wouldn't have done'

(Mrs AE, aged 72).

A letter to the *British Medical Journal* pleaded for a return to home births, because women in hospital were left alone 'to get on with it'. (Hutton 1945). Women interviewed in the 1946 survey complained of being left on their own in labour-rooms, even in the second stage (Joint Committee 1948). The Maternity Services Committee (Ministry of Health 1959) heard evidence from several witnesses that 'women were left too long alone in labour, some ascribing this to shortage of staff, others to lack of understanding'. The 'general complaint that there was in many hospitals too little regard for the personal dignity and emotional condition of women during pregnancy and childbirth' was investigated by the Central Health Services Council (1961). They found that 'loneliness seems to be the chief cause of dissatisfaction'. They dismissed the work of Grantly Dick Read, because 'much of his success in conducting confinements was due to his personal presence throughout the whole of labour and his respect for the emotional needs of the expectant mother and father'.

Instead of considering the value of a supportive presence and respect for emotional needs in alleviating the anguish of loneliness, the Council demonstrated a rather strange perception of the kind of company needed by a labouring woman. Of the average 16 hours of a primigravida's first stage, they said: 'A large part of this may be spent in the labour ward or first stage room with very few people to talk to and very little to do.' Staff might have 'no time or little inclination to spend time in chatting with her'. Again they could have considered Read's words on the 'irritations that intensify pain': 'How many nurses and doctors realise the agony of conversation, often about ill-chosen topics? There are awful people who try to cheer their patients by bright remarks. The mind should be rested, and some measure of pain will be spared' (Read 1943).

These reports also indicate that the loneliness women complained of in the 1940s and 1950s was exacerbated by not knowing what was happening to them and, for some, not being believed when they said their baby was about to be born. It was not just ignorance that resulted in women delivering unaided. Some were treated so rudely that they were afraid to ring the bell again (Central Health Services Council 1961).

The constant witnessing of pain, coupled with autocratic and largely unsupervised control over a stream of frightened, possibly unduly nervous, but utterly defenceless women, separated from their husbands and friends at their most critical moment, is perhaps not conducive to a sympathetic attitude of mind on the part of the labour-ward staff ...

(National Birthday Trust Fund 1956)

This extract is taken from evidence presented to the Maternity Services Committee. The submission also refers to many letters of protest at the way some hospital midwives treated women in labour. An eminent obstetrician (Morris 1960) quoted from letters received by a weekly women's journal about their experiences in hospital, and concluded that 'the feeling of personal achievement is lost, drowned in a sea of inhumanity'. He asked: '... do some nurses and doctors find childbirth repugnant and not something rather wonderful?'.

It is interesting that even in the 1950s it was suggested that staffing clinical areas rather than women—discontinuity of care—resulted in women losing the opportunity to receive appropriate, sensitive, individualised care during labour. The National Birthday Trust Fund feared that 'those women willing to enter upon a career of endless labour-ward duty might be particularly hard-natured types of women, callous to the sufferings of their patients'. Whether they were 'hard-natured' to begin with, or whether indifference was cultivated as a coping mechanism, it is certain that midwives working exclusively on a labour ward did in fact lose 'the opportunity to think of the mother as a woman and not merely as a case' (National Birthday Trust Fund 1956).

The fear of the unknown referred to earlier would be intensified not only by loneliness and staff attitudes, but by the surroundings themselves and by hearing the cries of other terrified women in labour. Another British Medical Journal correspondence highlighted the effects of the hospital environment and communal labour wards on the 'chaotic ignorance in which many women are still allowed to approach their first confinement' (Egerton 1948). Open first stage rooms were common, and even privacy for delivery was not guaranteed. It is difficult to believe that practising relaxation while imagining lying on a lawn under a tree could adequately prepare a woman for such an experience.

The contrast with giving birth at home was stark—even if the midwife could not be there throughout, the woman was not alone, and she was the only person in labour. She was 'the centre of attraction' (Ministry of Health 1959). Mrs FS, aged 80, remembers waiting for labour to start after her membranes had ruptured:

'They bound me up, very, very tight. Like a pole on the … well it was wrapped up in wool or something on the side of me, then a very wide bandage, and rolled it round and round me. So then they put me to bed and left me, and it was pouring with rain, and I thought, "Help! if this is having a baby, I'm not going to have another one. And if I do have another one, I'm going to have it at home, because nobody knows what I'm going through, you know." Because I was scared. I wasn't really in any pain.'

The staff shortages of the time are recognised, but it must be concluded that no need was perceived to mitigate the frightening effects of the hospital environment by supportive companionship. Women labouring in hospital were expected to get on with it on their own, and this expectation remained in the culture of many hospitals for decades. The suggestion that (probably equally frightened) husbands should be allowed to visit (Central Health Services Council 1961) can be interpreted as evading the fundamental issue of the role of the midwife.

Midwifery textbooks meanwhile stressed that a woman should never be left alone, emphasising the importance of her mental state, and the attitude of her attendant. 'Throughout this whole stage—the longest part of a labour—the midwife's kindliness, firmness, and patience may well be tested. Her reward comes as she sees her patient retaining her self-confidence and responding to encouragement' (Johnstone 1946). Various measures are suggested to help women cope with pain, such as activity, change of position, mobilisation, distraction, companionship, sacral pressure and massage. Any sedation or analgesia that may be needed takes second place. The earlier editions of Myles' *A textbook for midwives* placed considerable emphasis on the emotional, supportive aspects of care in labour, though the woman's role is portrayed as more passive and dependent on the midwife for the 'patient, almost maternal, care and companionship' she desires and needs (Myles 1961). In subsequent editions the psychological considerations are given progressively less attention, and available drugs become correspondingly more important. As an anaesthetist commented (Roberts 1950): 'midwives are taught that during the early part of labour patients should be kept as active as conditions permit, and that they should be encouraged to take light diet and to drink as much as possible. How are they to do these things if attempts are made to lay the patients low with analgesic drugs?'

BIRTH EXPERIENCES AND THE IMPORTANCE OF MEMORIES

The Working Party on Midwives (Ministry of Health 1949) believed that the lack of effective pain relief available in the community was responsible for increasing numbers of women choosing to give birth in hospital. Subsequent analyses have agreed that this was at least part of the explanation (Lewis 1980). From the evidence presented here, there was clearly a dramatic increase in the use of sedative and analgesic drugs, but this appears as likely to have been the result as it was to have been the cause of women being in hospital.

It has been suggested that 'it may be more important to reduce the affective component of labour pain than to reduce its intensity' (Niven & Gijsbers 1984), but instead of considering the part played by fear and anxiety in women's distress, midwives in the 1940s and 1950s turned increasingly to drugs as a first resort. Meanwhile, procedures were taught during pregnancy which offered a woman who wanted it the opportunity to cope with her labour and give birth fully awake and aware. Midwives undermined the message in the classes by implying that it was not achievable (or perhaps even desirable), and finally sabotaged it during labour by leaving her alone for long periods. This was made possible by the administration of drugs which not only rendered the woman muzzy and disorientated, but were also potentially harmful to her baby. Marjorie Tew (1995) has argued that obstetric interventions in the 1960s and 1970s resulted in midwives giving more attention to machinery than to supporting women in labour, but it seems that midwives' interest had already turned away from their traditional role. The identification of only advanced labour as 'real work', as suggested by Hunt & Symonds (1995), may actually have been a feature of hospital practice for a considerable time.

There is evidence that women experiencing the most aggressively managed labours may require little analgesia if they are guaranteed constant personal attention (O'Driscoll & Meagher 1980). For many women, supportive care is more important than any other intervention (Shields 1978, Morgan et al 1984, Niven 1994), and a number of studies suggest that companionship can actually enable women to labour and give birth more effectively and with better outcomes for themselves and their babies (see, for example, Sosa et al 1980, Klaus et al 1986, Hofmeyr et al 1991, Kennell et al 1991).

Measurable benefits are useful for arguing a case, but the obsession with scientifically acceptable evidence should not outweigh the importance of the subjective element. A woman's concern for qualitative aspects of the birth experience is not an indulgence. The way she is treated, whether her autonomy is respected, how her concept of herself is affected by her performance, all leave indelible impressions. Expectations are formed by many factors (see Green et al 1990); but it is likely that a woman's intended strategies for coping with labour are those which she hopes will enable her to survive the process with her self-esteem intact, whether this involves the use of drugs or not. Whatever the outcome, she will relive the birth again and again, searching for explanations, trying to make sense of what happened and integrating the experience into her life story.

SUMMARY

Many of the women interviewed for the present study are still deeply moved by their experiences of 50 or 60 years ago. Penny Simkin's (1991, 1992) research confirmed that women's memories remain vivid and emotional for many years, as well as startlingly accurate. She concluded: 'it is clear that the birth experience has a powerful effect on women with a potential for permanent or long-term positive or negative impact' (Simkin 1991). We need to be constantly aware that anything we say or do may be remembered by a woman for the rest of her life, and that the way we make her feel about herself may change her

life. If we are committed to providing care which is truly woman-centred, rather than, yet again, what attendants think is best, our prime concern must be to enable every woman to emerge as victor rather than victim (Oakley 1980) from her birth experiences.

REFERENCES

Allied Newspapers Ltd (undated, c. 1920) The complete medical encyclopedia and household doctor. Allied Newspapers, London

Beinart J 1990 Obstetric analgesia and the control of childbirth in twentieth century Britain. In: Garcia J, Kilpatrick R, Richards M (eds) The politics of maternity care: services for childbearing women in twentieth century Britain. Clarendon, Oxford

Billewicz-Driemel A M, Milne M D 1976 Long term assessment of extradural analgesia for the relief of pain in labour II. Sense of 'deprivation' after extradural analgesia in labour: relevant or not? British Journal of Anaesthesia 48: 139–144

Bluff R, Holloway I 1994 'They know best': women's perceptions of midwifery care during labour and childbirth. Midwifery 10: 157–164

British Medical Journal 1934 Report of the Liverpool Medical Institution. 1: 3819, 17th March: 501–502

Brook D 1976 Naturebirth: preparing for natural birth in an age of technology. Penguin, Harmondsworth

Brown R C, Fraser D, Dobbs R H 1962 Midwifery: principles and practice for pupil midwives, 5th edn. Edward Arnold, London

Browne F J 1944 Antenatal and postnatal care, 5th edn. J & A Churchill, London

Central Council for Health Education 1957 Where mothers learn. Health Education Journal XV(4): 216–222

Central Health Services Council Standing Maternity and Midwifery Advisory Committee 1961 Human relations in obstetrics. HMSO, London

Close S 1980 Birth report: extracts from over 4000 personal experiences. NFER Publishing, Windsor

Clyne D G W 1963 A textbook of gynaecology and obstetrics. Longmans, London

Copstick S, Hayes R W, Taylor K E, Morris N F 1985 A test of a common assumption regarding the use of antenatal training during labour. Journal of Psychosomatic Research 29(2): 215–218

Copstick S M, Taylor K E, Hayes R, Morris N 1986 Partner support and the use of coping techniques in labour. Journal of Psychosomatic Research 30(4): 497–503

Cosslett T 1994 Women writing childbirth: modern discourses of motherhood. Manchester University Press, Manchester

Crawford J S 1972 The second thousand epidural blocks in an obstetric hospital practice. British Journal of Anaesthesia 44: 1277–1286

Crawford J S 1984 Obstetric analgesia and anaesthesia, 2nd edn. Churchill Livingstone, Edinburgh

Da Cruz V 1967 Mayes' handbook for midwives, 7th edn. Bailliere, Tindall & Cassell, London

Egerton M E 1948 Letter. British Medical Journal 1(4556): 903

Fairbairn J S 1918 A text-book for midwives. Oxford University Press, London

Fairbairn J S 1944 Constructive, educational and social aspects of antenatal care. In: Browne F J (ed) Antenatal and postnatal care, 5th edn. J & A Churchill, London

Green J M 1993 Expectations and experiences of pain in labour: findings from a large prospective study. Birth 20(2): 65–72

Green J M, Coupland V A, Kitzinger J V 1990 Expectations, experiences, and psychological outcomes of childbirth: a prospective study of 825 women. Birth 17(1): 15–24

Heardman H 1958 Relaxation and exercise for natural childbirth. E & S Livingstone, Edinburgh

Heardman H 1973 A way to natural childbirth. A manual for physiotherapists and parents-to-be, 3rd edn (revised and re-edited by Maria Ebner). Churchill Livingstone, Edinburgh

Hofmeyr G J, Nikidom V C, Wolman W-L, Chalmers B E, Kramer T 1991 Companionship to modify the clinical birth environment: effects on progress and perceptions of labour, and breastfeeding. British Journal of Obstetrics and Gynaecology 98: 756–764

Hunt S, Symonds A 1995 The social meaning of midwifery. Macmillan, Basingstoke

Hutton L 1945 Letter. British Medical Journal 1(4400): 639

Johnstone R W 1946 The midwife's text-book of the principles and practice of midwifery, 2nd edn. Adam & Charles Black, London

Johnstone R W 1962 The midwife's text-book of the principles and practice of midwifery, 8th edn. Adam & Charles Black, London

Joint Committee of the Royal College of Obstetricians and Gynaecologists and the Population Investigation Committee 1948 Maternity in Great Britain. Oxford University Press, London

Karmel M 1965 Thank you, Dr Lamaze: a mother's experiences in painless childbirth. Dolphin Books, Garden City, NY

Kennell J, Klaus M, McGrath S, Robertson S, Hinkley C 1991 Continuous emotional support during labor in a US hospital: a randomised controlled trial. Journal of the American Medical Association 265(17): 2197–2201

Kitzinger S 1967 The experience of childbirth. Penguin, Harmondsworth

Kitzinger J 1990 Strategies of the early childbirth movement: a casestudy of the National Childbirth Trust. In: Garcia J, Kilpatrick R, Richards M (eds) The politics of maternity care: services for childbearing women in twentieth century Britain. Clarendon, Oxford

Klaus M H, Kennell J H, Robertson S S, Sosa R 1986 Effects of social support during parturition on maternal and infant morbidity. British Medical Journal 293(6547): 585–587

Lewis J 1980 The politics of motherhood: child and maternal welfare in England 1900–1939. Croom Helm, London

Madders J 1958 Before and after childbirth: exercises and relaxation, 2nd edn. E & S Livingstone, Edinburgh

Ministry of Health 1949 Report of the Working Party on Midwives. HMSO, London

Ministry of Heath 1959 Report of the Maternity Services Committee. HMSO, London

Morgan B M, Bulpitt C J, Clifton P, Lewis P J 1984 The consumers' attitude to obstetric care. British Journal of Obstetrics and Gynaecology 19(7): 624–628

Morris N 1960 Human relations in obstetric practice. Lancet 7130: 913–915

Myles M F 1956 A textbook for midwives, 2nd edn. E & S Livingstone, Edinburgh

Myles M F 1961 A textbook for midwives, 4th edn. E & S Livingstone, Edinburgh

Myles M F 1968 A textbook for midwives, 6th edn. E & S Livingstone, Edinburgh

Myles M F 1975 Textbook for midwives with modern concepts of obstetric and neonatal care, 8th edn. Churchill Livingstone, Edinburgh

National Birthday Trust Fund 1956 Extracts from evidence submitted to the Maternity Services (Cranbrook) Committee. Annexe 'F' in Report of the Maternity Services Emergency Informal Committee 1963

Niven C 1994 Coping with labour pain: the midwife's role. In: Robinson S, Thomson A M (eds) Midwives, research and childbirth, vol III. Chapman & Hall, London

Niven C, Gijsbers K 1984 Obstetric and non-obstetric factors related to labour pain. Journal of Reproductive and Infant Psychology 2: 61–78

Oakley A 1980 Women confined: towards a sociology of childbirth. Martin Robertson, Oxford

O'Driscoll K 1975 An obstetrician's view of pain. British Journal of Anaesthesia 48: 139–144

O'Driscoll K, Meagher D 1980 Active management of labour. W B Saunders, London

Read G D 1943 Revelation of childbirth: the principles and practice of natural childbirth, 2nd edn. William Heinemann, London

Read G D 1950 Introduction to motherhood. William Heinemann, London

Read G D 1959 Childbirth without fear: the principles and practice of natural childbirth. First Perennial Library edition (1970). Harper & Row, New York

Roberts H 1950 Letter. British Medical Journal 1(4652): 551

Shields D 1978 Nursing care in labour and patient satisfaction: a descriptive study. Journal of Advanced Nursing 3(6): 535–550

Simkin P 1991 Just another day in a woman's life? Women's long-term perceptions of their first birth experience: Part I. Birth 18(4): 203–210

Simkin P 1992 Just another day in a woman's life? Part II: nature and consistency of women's long-term memories of their first birth experiences. Birth 19(2): 64–81

Sosa R, Kennell J, Klaus M, Robertson S, Urrutia J 1980 The effect of a supportive companion on perinatal problems, length of labour and mother-infant interaction. New England Journal of Medicine 303(11): 597–600

Tew M 1995 Safer childbirth? a critical history of maternity care, 2nd edn. Chapman & Hall, London

Vaughan K 1951 Exercises before childbirth. Faber & Faber, London

6

A cultural experience of pain

Linda Hayes

LEARNING OUTCOMES

At the end of this chapter the reader will have

- **an introduction to the cultural influences on pain perception**

- **identified some of the issues relating to the experiences of women from a particular ethnic group**

- **considered the significance of effective communication on understanding and management of pain in labour for ethnic minority groups**

- **identified some key considerations for midwifery practice and increased cultural awareness.**

Ideas about health and illness are determined by the society in which we live. There are wide differences in the perceptions of health both within a single culture and from one culture to another. How people accept and react to health, prevention of illness and treatment are as much a part of culture as language, religion, family patterns and behaviour. In each culture there is a way of life within which an individual may acquire attitudes, values, beliefs and their religious teachings, which may in turn bear an influence on responses to pain, fear and other emotional sensations. According to Melzack (1973) pain is a sensation perceived by the individual, the intensity of and response to which is affected by culture, previous experience of pain, emotional state and anticipation.

In many cultures, childbirth and parturition are considered to be secretive matters to be hidden from view and not discussed. It is hardly surprising that for women who have limited opportunity for verbal interaction outside their own social group that myths associated with childbirth abound. A consequence of this is that many women are still ignorant of the process of parturition, and because of racial myths and overheard whispers, they have acquired a 'conditioned reflex' in which childbirth is associated with pain, distress and fear of the unknown.

Despite there being more second and third generation Asians in Britain, communication is still a major problem faced by such ethnic groups (Hayes 1989, unpubl. data). If health workers cannot effectively communicate with those they assist and care for, they will be unable to identify needs, agree on mutually acceptable care and generally promote health education. Consequently, Asian women not fluent in English may be unable to make their needs known, and therefore those needs could go unmet, causing frustration, reducing standards of care and creating inequality.

For the purposes of this chapter, Asian women are defined as those whose family originated from the Indian subcontinent. This definition embraces those women who were born in the UK as well as those who have come to the UK from India, Pakistan and Bangladesh and distinguishes them from other women (e.g. of Chinese origin) who could also be called Asian. This chapter will discuss the assertion often quoted by health professionals that Asian childbearing women have a 'low pain threshold'. In responding to individual needs of women, midwives should acknowledge that the manifestation of pain will be influenced by cultural experience, and therefore must avoid holding preconceived ideas about pain expression and subsequent management.

EFFECTIVE COMMUNICATION

Understanding what is available and making the right choice can be daunting for anyone, but especially for those whose first language is not English. For ethnic minority women the maternity services have been described as inappropriate, inaccessible and inadequate (National Association of Health Authorities 1990). Individuals from ethnic minority communities have life styles, family patterns, religious beliefs, dietary norms, expectations and priorities that differ significantly from those of the indigenous population. Health service personnel continue to be singled out for criticism. Yet another report acknowledges that the problems of communication significantly affect the opportunity to make informed choices about health care. The report (House of Commons Health Services Committee 1992) clearly states that 'the transfer of information depends on successful communication to all women. Choices for women who do not share the same language and culture as the providers must be enhanced through training and well resourced interpreters, advocates and link workers.'

A woman whose health advisors cannot speak her language is not only likely to be lonely and confused; there is also a danger that she will not be properly treated. Without comprehensive information on maternity health services, in an appropriate language and medium, women are ill-equipped to make informed choices about investigative procedures and other services available to them. They are consequently ill-equipped to make informed choices about pain relief in labour. So it must be the responsibility of the health services to ensure that proper communication is possible. Standard 1 of the *Patient's Charter* (Department of Health 1991) has exhorted all providers of care to show 'respect for privacy, dignity and religious and cultural beliefs'.

PROVISION OF MATERNITY CARE

The current trend towards care within the community, especially associated with childbirth, potentially has the advantage of women being cared for within their own family and cultural environment, thereby enabling them to take advantage of the customs and traditions surrounding the parturient women. Each culture values its traditions, beliefs and customs; they offer a sense of identity, security and cohesion to minority communities in a predominantly individualistic secular society. Whereas first generation Asians who have settled here feel the need to affirm their cultural values, the second generation Asians are often torn between the two cultures.

The 1991 census identified that there is an estimated three million people of ethnic minority origin residing in England and Wales, constituting 6% of the total population. However, their distribution is uneven, accounting for up to 60% of the population in some areas (Balarajan & Raleigh 1992). The NHS provides a diverse range of health care services, however it has been slow in recognising the demographic changes that have taken place over time. The service provision and delivery of care is often based on a white culture-specific approach, dealing primarily with the needs of the indigenous white population.

The Black report (Townsend & Davidson 1988) and *The health divide* (Whitehead 1987) have suggested that the NHS does not provide a comparable level of service to all social classes and ethnic groups, with the white middle classes deriving maximum benefit from health care provision. Because Britain is a multiracial, multicultural society, health workers, and midwives in particular, need to be prepared to work with clients from various backgrounds, and to present health care in ways that are appropriate to each client.

More than a decade has passed and evidence suggests that inequalities in health service provision and access continue. The health of ethnic minorities is discussed at length in a report of the Chief Medical Officer (Department of Health 1992), which pointed out that 'the NHS must address the particular needs of the black and ethnic minorities living in this country, and take positive steps to eliminate discrimination'.

STEREOTYPICAL VIEWS

Stereotyping, in this context, involves a lack of recognition of the many differences amongst individuals from certain cultural and ethnic groups. An area which often stimulates such stereotyping, is that associated with some of the cultural practices related to childbirth, since they differ from those regarded as 'normal' or

desirable in this country. Henley (1979), for example, discusses the custom of Asian women staying in bed with their baby for some days after the birth, when they are usually given special foods and taken care of by a midwife and female relatives, in order to allow mothers to rest and regain their strength. Similarly, Woollett & Dosanjh-Matwala (1990) explored the views of 32 Asian women living in East London about their experiences of childbirth. This study identified that this group of Asian women viewed the opportunity to rest and recover postnatally as more central to their care than did the hospitals.

A number of researchers, notably Henley (1979) and more recently Mares et al (1985), have specifically provided a wealth of ethnic and cultural information that should be of value in helping health professionals to tailor midwifery care and advice in order to make it as culturally acceptable and relevant as possible. However, a small-scale ethnographic study undertaken by Bowler (1993), which investigated the delivery of maternity care to patients of south-Asian descent, maintained that some midwives hold stereotypical views that call into question equity of care. This paper examined the stereotypes held by midwives in one British hospital of women of south-Asian descent. The midwives' stereotype contained four main themes:

- difficulty in communicating with the women
- women's lack of compliance with the care available and their abuse of the service
- a tendency to 'make a fuss about nothing'
- a lack of a 'normal maternal instinct'.

Women with little English were branded 'rude and unintelligent' and were subsequently unable to form a relationship with the midwives or challenge any misconceptions. Some of the midwives questioned expressed the view that language difficulties are the 'patients' problem' and that 'they should learn English'. These commonly held attitudes and beliefs may therefore be interpreted as 'victim blaming', an issue which needs to be overcome by all providers of health care. *The Patient's Charter* (Department of Health 1991) states that the health service should set standards which aim for 'respect for privacy, dignity and religious and cultural beliefs and arrangements to ensure everyone, including those with special needs can use the service'.

Bonaparte (1979) argued that a potentially therapeutic relationship between the nurse and a client may be handicapped by the tendency for the nurse to have ethnocentric beliefs about the superiority of Western health standards. The findings of this study indicate that there is little apparent understanding by respondents of the illness behaviour of certain clients, and that some respondents were ethnocentric in their interpretation of the clients' and their relatives' behaviour, particularly their perceptions relating to the aspects of a 'sick role', seen as 'taking to their beds', or clients' preferences for particular types of food, prepared and brought to them in hospital.

In a study conducted by Murphy & Macleod Clark (1993), data were collected through a process of in-depth interviews with 18 trained nurses. Some of the respondents appeared to accept the inevitability of poor communication and did nothing to improve it. It is difficult to find an explanation for this. Forrest (1989) found that, when clients are deemed hard to care for, nurses may experience feelings of negativity, may distance themselves from the client, and may limit themselves to giving 'physical' or 'routine' care.

Distortion of black culture, blaming the culture for medical problems, and placing priority on changing that culture rather than changing the practices of existing institutions, have become important characteristics of the operation of medical institutions. In 1981, the Brent Community Health Council published a report entitled *Black people and the Health Service*, in which this process was discussed. The authors quote a group of GPs in Brent who said that 'the pain threshold for Asians is half that of Caucasians ... they complain twice as much for half the reason ... they come with minor symptoms' (Brent Community Health Council 1981). The report identified that it was natural for the 'sick' to express suffering and anxiety, and that Asian patients may moan and cry in a way that upsets others around them.

Every individual is an amalgam of their sociological and psychological background. The influence of childhood experience and the beliefs to which they have been culturally exposed will in turn influence the perception and experience of pain sensation. A person who has, for example, been brought up throughout childhood to believe that they must 'grin and bear it' will perceive pain very differently to another who experiences what may initially be outwardly perceived as a similar painful event. This person may have been socialised into believing that they are able to express their feelings and sensations openly, often vocally and vociferously. Such attitudes will pervade adult life, often giving rise to the stereotypical views of certain cultural groups who openly express pain, or alternatively maintain a 'stiff upper lip'.

Women in labour from various cultural backgrounds, may therefore vocalise their pain more readily. It is perhaps ethnocentric views—that, for example, everyone must 'grin and bear it', or that 'they all make a lot of noise'—which will inevitably lead to prejudice and discrimination. In gathering information and evidence towards the review of policy in the NHS, The Expert Maternity Group took measures to obtain the views of women who are not associated with any particular group or organisation. These included surveys of mothers from Asian and Afro-Caribbean origins. One expert's views are an illustration of some unhelpful generalisations: 'Carol Baxter, a health and race consultant ... emphasised that variations between individuals within ethnic and social groups may be as wide as those between the groups themselves ... the preference of individuals should always be sought and respected' (Department of Health 1993).

A CULTURE OF PAIN

Helman (1990) makes a distinction between 'private' and 'public' pain, suggesting that reactions to pain are not simply involuntary or instinctual, but take place within a social context and contain a voluntary component. Individuals may or may not take action to relieve pain, and the help of others may or may not be enlisted. Certain cultural or social groups may value stoicism; in the face of pain each cultural group has its own unique language of distress. Hence, keeping pain private, or expressing it publicly, may be either desirable or undesirable when viewed within the context of a particular social group's beliefs and value systems. Moreover, cultural beliefs and values may serve to 'normalise' experiences of pain which for others may appear problematic. However, a conflict frequently emerges when care attendant and client do not share the same language or culture.

Wright (1983) undertook a survey of GPs based in an area of Newcastle which had a high population of people from Pakistan. Women from this community spoke little English and according to the doctors often presented with 'trivial complaints'. The doctors initially regarded these women as nuisances and presumably conveyed as much to them, yet when the language barriers were removed by the presence of an interpreter or a doctor who could speak the same language, the doctors' attitudes changed and these so-called trivial complaints disappeared.

The definition of pain, just like definitions of health and illness, is culturally determined (Ludwig-Beymer 1989). According to Meinhart & McCaffrey (1983) cultural expectations may specify:

- different reactions according to age, sex, and occupation
- what treatment to seek
- the intensity and duration of pain that should be tolerated
- what responses should be made
- who to report to when pain occurs
- what types of pain requires attention.

CULTURE AND LABOUR

Weisenberg & Caspi (1989) examined the effects of sociocultural, family of origin and educational influences on the verbal ratings of pain and pain behaviour during childbirth. It was found that women of Middle-Eastern origin gave higher ratings of pain and demonstrated more pain behaviour, as compared with women from a Western background. This was especially associated with those Middle-Eastern women of a low educational background. The authors concluded

from this study that 'sociocultural group of origin, as well as educational background, are important in determining pain perception and behaviour'. The study identifies the importance of such knowledge in preparing women appropriately for childbirth. Actually to compare specific cultural groups can be seen as prejudicial in itself; the uniqueness of each culture must therefore always be acknowledged.

Alibhai (1988) studied the effect of prejudice and racism on black and Asian women. The author described how not being white was detrimental to the type of care these women received. On an individual level a degree of racism was encountered in the attitude of some midwives. Their generalisations that black women deliver easily and Asian women have low pain thresholds was shown to lead to their pain being treated less seriously, and to white women being more likely to be offered analgesia.

Midwives must be able to communicate with those they support in labour if they are to identify needs, agree on mutually acceptable care and generally promote health education. However, care throughout pregnancy and childbirth remains strongly service-oriented. It was evident from a study conducted by Hayes (1989, unpubl. data) that little attempt is made to build upon, or indeed acknowledge, the competence of interpreters/linkworkers, which could ultimately provide better understanding between health professionals and Asian women throughout pregnancy. Many difficulties and tensions in the interactions between health care professionals were demonstrated.

It was apparent at times that the health professionals had no clear understanding of the range of Asian languages spoken by the population. Furthermore, direct translation of English into an Asian language is not always possible or appropriate. In addition, it emerged that there was difficulty in 'representing' both health professionals and the women. In practice the role of the interpreter/linkworker was defined by the health professional to whom she was accountable, and only secondly by the woman—a practice which therefore minimises opportunities for the woman to have any choice or control in her care. In essence the interpreters/linkworkers were an invaluable resource, but essentially an invisible asset. Their absence at times outside 'normal working hours' (i.e. '9-to-5') was a cause for concern. This often resulted in requests being made for assistance with translation by a variety of people. As well as family members, junior hospital doctors or ancillary workers were utilised for interpreting women's needs in labour, a factor which often caused distress and confusion at times when every attempt should be made to avoid it.

The report of the Expert Maternity Group (Department of Health 1993), *Changing Childbirth*, recommends the use of 'well resourced interpreters, advocates and linkworkers' to overcome language barriers and enable women from ethnic minorities to have the same opportunities as other women, yet for a long time women have been expected to provide their own interpreters by bringing along partners, friends or even children to interpret for them. This practice has been strongly criticised as unsatisfactory, and *The race relations code of practice in maternity services* (Department of Health 1994a) refers to this practice as inappropriate or even dangerous as it leads to misunderstandings and overlooks cultural differences which may inhibit women from discussing sensitive and intimate matters in front of others.

Of all the services provided by the NHS, maternity care, and care in labour in particular, should be provided in such a way that women and their families feel comfortable and at ease. Any alienation, especially if racially or culturally based, will further disadvantage a group of women within our society who already experience unequal access to maternity services. The failure to take up antenatal care is recognised in Short (1980, 1984), and yet since that time relatively little appears to have been done to address this issue.

Good maternity care requires intimate and sensitive communication between women and those who care for them. A woman who is cared for in labour by midwives who cannot speak her language is not only likely to be lonely and confused, but there is also a potential for her treatment to be inadequate. It is therefore the responsibility of health care professionals and the health services to ensure that effective communication is possible. By providing training for those working with women for whom English is a second language and introducing policies to positively recruit staff who speak relevant languages, health authorities would be recognising their obligation to meet the needs of the whole community. While some improvements require additional resources, much could be done by imaginative and sensitive adaptations to current services, and by ensuring that NHS employment and training stress a commitment to racial equality.

The care women receive in labour remains strongly service-oriented amongst health professionals. Little attempt is made to build on or indeed acknowledge the lay competence of interpreters/linkworkers which could add to a better cultural understanding between health professionals and pregnant Asian women in their care. The problem of communicating with non-English speaking patients is characterised by half-hearted stop-gap measures. In this way the system just 'gets by' and is consequently a completely unsatisfactory situation for all concerned. All those caring for women in labour should be reminded that 'more research is needed on the choices that are important to different groups of women, there is no doubt that more advocates and linkworkers, better training and greater efforts to develop services in consultation with users will help' (House of Commons Health Services Committee 1992).

Having a baby in hospital can be a bewildering experience for any woman, but for someone who speaks little or no English it can make it particularly difficult to cope with effectively. Pregnancy and labour and birth are overwhelming experiences; it can be extremely frightening when birth takes place in a country where the culture and the language are both unfamiliar. Indeed, even women who have a good command of spoken English may not be able to cope with the specialised vocabulary of the health service. In particular, the terminology of analgesia/anaesthesia can be extremely perplexing and incomprehensible, especially when the labouring woman is frightened, in pain, tired and under stress. Those women with even a limited command of English may find that understanding of the language disappears at these times.

McGee (1993) poses a challenge to health professionals when, writing in a recent editorial, she claims that there is 'little evidence of any deep understanding of, or sensitivity towards, the diverse cultures and beliefs that make up our society'. The author further claims that 'nurses are tackling isolated issues rather than examining the underlying values and attitudes that pervade the provision of health care'. It is further purported that nurses are 'applying a coat of gloss to a system that perpetuates inequality and which, it seems, will continue to do so'.

In order to enable consumers of maternity services to exercise choice and control over the care they receive, midwives together with other health professionals have an obligation to empower women. Empowerment of women is only a reality if they are fully informed through access to good quality and appropriate information. If ethnic minority clients are to receive individualised care, then an accurate assessment of client needs and problems must be made.

CULTURAL CONSIDERATIONS FOR MIDWIFERY PRACTICE

The following are steps that should be taken to ensure that cultural difference in itself does not result in inequality of care between cultures:

• There should be an extension of the roles of advocate, interpreter and linkworker provision in order to facilitate effective, accessible and acceptable care in pregnancy, labour and the postnatal period to women of Asian and other ethnic groups.
• Health educators should consider organising preparation for parenthood classes that include culturally appropriate health education programmes for women of ethnic minority groups.
• More training should be provided to assist health workers in dealing with the health needs of a multiracial community.
• Shift working or 'on-call' systems should be encouraged so that interpreters/linkworkers would be available over a 24-hour period, especially to cover labour wards and assist community

midwives when deliveries are booked to take place within the home.
• Records and documentation used by health workers should indicate the language spoken by the client, preferably the mother tongue, so that effective use can be made of the interpreters'/linkworkers' linguistic skills.
• User held notes, which include sections for noting religious and cultural needs, should be utilised in order to provide a basis for effective information and a more personal individualised service
• More leaflets need to be translated into other languages and include images presented in a way in which Asian women can relate, in order to empower them to make informed choices in relation to all aspects of care.
• Seminars on Asian cultures and their relevance to health, presented to nursing and midwifery staff by interpreters/linkworkers and other Asian health professionals, should be encouraged to take place on a regular basis, in an effort to promote cultural awareness.

SUMMARY

It is clear that language is not the only barrier that needs to be negotiated between different cultures. Differences in customs extend to differences in pain perception and vocalisation, and differences in postnatal expectations of care, among others. In dealing with women from ethnic minorities, it is important for the midwives from a different culture to be aware of these differences so that complete equality of care provision for all women can be achieved.

REFERENCES

Alibhai 1988 Can't they see I'm me? Nursing Times 82 (1): 56
Balarajan R, Raleigh V 1992 The ethnic populations of England and Wales: the 1991 census. Health Trends 24: 113–116
Bonaparte B H 1979 Ego defensiveness, open–closed mindedness, and nurses' attitude towards culturally different patients. Nursing Research 28 (30): 166–171
Bowler 1993 Stereotypes of women of Asian descent in midwifery: some evidence. Midwifery 9: 7–16.

Brent Community Health Council 1981 Black people and the health service. Russell Press, Nottingham

Department of Health 1991 The Patient's Charter. HMSO, London

Department of Health 1992 On the state of the public health. HMSO, London.

Department of Health 1993 Report of the Expert Maternity Group – Changing childbirth. HMSO, London

Department of Health 1994a The race relations code of practice in maternity services. HMSO, London

Department of Health 1994b Maternity Services for Asian Women. NHS Management Executive, HMSO, London.

Forrest D 1989 The experience of caring. Journal of Advanced Nursing 14: 815–823

Helman C 1990 Culture, health and illness, 2nd edn. Butterworth Heinemann, Oxford

Henley A 1979 Asian patients in hospital and at home. King Edward's Hospital Fund for London, London

House of Commons Health Services Committee 1992 Second report. Maternity Services, vol 1. HMSO, London

Ludwig-Beymer P 1989 Transcultural aspects of pain. In: Boyle J S, Andrews M M (eds) Transcultural concepts in nursing care. Scott–Foresman, Glenview, Illinois

McGee P 1993 Does racism exist in nursing? British Journal of Nursing 2 (16): 791

Mares P, Henley A, Baxter C 1985 Health care in a multi–racial Britain. Health Education Council and National Extension College, Cambridge

Meinhart N T, McCaffery M 1983 Pain: a nursing approach to assessment and analysis. Appleton Century Crofts, Norwalk, Conneticut

Melzack R D 1973 The puzzle of pain. Basic Books, New York

Murphy K, McCleod Clark J 1993 Nurses experiences of caring for ethnic-minority clients. Journal of Advanced Nursing 18: 442–450

National Association of Health Authorities 1990 Review of services for black and ethnic minority people. Maternity Services Bulletin No 2. NAHA, Birmingham

Short R 1980 Second report from the Social Services Committee, session 1979–80, Perinatal and neonatal mortality. HMSO, London

Short R 1984 Third report from the Social Services Committee, session 1983–84, Perinatal and neonatal mortality. HMSO, London

Townsend P, Davidson N 1988 Inequalities in health. Penguin Books, London

Weisenberg M, Caspi Z 1989 Cultural and educational influences on pain of childbirth. Journal of Pain and Symptom Management 4 (1): 13–19

Whitehead M 1987 The health divide: inequalities in health in the 1990s. Health Education Publications, London.

Woolett A, Dosanjh-Matwala N 1990 Postnatal care: the attitudes and experiences of Asian women in east London. Midwifery 6: 178–184

Wright C M 1983 Language and communication problems in the Asian community. Journal of the Royal College of General Practitioners 33: 101–104

7

Care by midwives: women's experiences

Lesley Choucri

LEARNING OUTCOMES

At the end of this chapter the reader will have

- **an introduction to an area of research into the care given by midwives to women in labour**

- **explored some women's actual experiences of care by midwives and the effect on their perception of labour**

- **identified some of the main themes influencing the 'mastery' of birth**

- **explored the interaction between the woman in labour and her midwife**

- **reflected on the influence of midwifery care on labour, pain perception and relief of pain.**

Birth has a special social and emotional significance for women and their partners; it is a life event, a human experience. Midwives sit with women through hours of labour, spending time and energy to provide care—a constant companion. I am one of those midwives. I am also a woman and a mother, and it became increasingly important to me to relate the study presented in this chapter to midwifery practice and to women's lived experiences of labour, pain and birth. I wished to hear and share what women knew, the 'truth' as they saw it; in the process hoping to help us as midwives to develop an understanding of behaviour that will enable us to provide care which is valued and of use to the women we serve.

With these thoughts uppermost in my mind, I utilised a phenomenological approach to the gathering and analysis of data about women's experiences of care by midwives. Such an approach involves understanding people in terms of the way in which they exist in the world as beings grounded in everyday life, and 'provides a lens through which we may focus on the nature of the lived experience' (Darbyshire 1994). For the purpose of this study, the focus is upon midwives, labour, pain and birth, as expressed from the woman's viewpoint.

Using a qualitative methodology allowed a group of women to be subjective about their life experience, and hence the results are contextual and cannot be generalised to other situations. The methodology attends to the nature of shared practices and common meanings, and its aim is not to provide answers to questions but rather to gather information on human experience. Such methods give the women's perspective of the social and cultural meanings of the midwifery care system which they have to negotiate to receive care from professionals. The findings are therefore descriptive rather than explanatory, the purpose being to improve the knowledge base of midwives who provide care.

Women's subjectivity of their experiences of pain in childbirth and care in the hands of the midwives is the essence of this work, which was undertaken in 1993, and the women in the study are to be thanked, as they were trusting enough to give their testimonies to me, a stranger and a midwife within the institution where they were receiving care. It was a privilege that they felt able to share their stories with me and perhaps in the telling, we as midwives can know their knowing. As Graham (1983) reminds us, much of midwifery care during labour and birth goes on behind closed doors, unseen and not spoken about. It is perhaps only through this phenomenological approach that we may share some of this knowledge, by the telling of women's experiences, and thereby value the women we care for.

Seven women agreed to participate in taped interviews. The small number of women is an important issue within the study for two essential reasons. Firstly, interviews produce many words which then have be transcribed and analysed—to increase the sample would have created an unmanageable amount of data and would thus have weakened the research. Secondly, in qualitative research, the best informant is one who has personal experience of the event in question and who can therefore express inner feelings as well as the physiological feelings which accompanied her experiences (Omery 1983). Thus to use a large random sample of all mothers would have been inappropriate. In the event, seven first time mothers were asked to participate, all of whom had a normal birth, attended by a midwife. All were selected because they had their own unique view of the phenomenon to be explored and were willing to share their knowledge.

During the interviews, the women talked freely about their birth experience and I discovered that they were eager to share their new self-knowledge. I also found that, through their disclosure, I as a midwife/researcher shared a sense of self-discovery concerning the nature of women and women as midwives. This supports Stanley's (1991) view of childbirth as a shared experience whereby we recognise ourselves in others and they recognise themselves in us, both parties thus being able to speak of common experiences grounded in individual knowing. As Joanne, a participant, stated: 'You want someone like yourself to look after you. I needed someone to say, "I know what you're going through".'

I transcribed all the data by hand and then analysed the information using Colaizzi's (1978) method in order to extract the emergent themes. The themes will be described alongside the supporting literature and the women's comments will be presented as spoken.

THE THEMES

Mastery of their birth: the women's perception of control during childbirth

The sense of mastery was key to a successful birth experience, and coping with the pain meant that the women could mobilise their inner resources to deal personally with these new mental and physical experiences. Mastery for this group of women meant having choices about what happened during the birth process, with the midwife supporting those choices and having respect for the decisions each woman had made about her care.

It is well documented that, in going into hospital to give birth, women are removed from their own source of power and support—their home—and often perceive the hospital as an institution where they have little influence over their own lives (Kirkham 1986, Murphy-Black 1995). They therefore expect to find a place with female experts who will help them and keep them safe (Raphael–Leff 1990). Mastery means taking responsibility for oneself, with the midwife giving help, no more and no less than needed, and respecting the woman as a person with the strength and confidence to give birth to her baby:

'You've got to feel something, if you don't you can't control it. She [the midwife] let me have the choice, she left it totally up to me. I wanted a bit of help, but I wanted to be in control.'

Harwood (1988), in her subjective account of her births in hospital, describes how she felt 'useless, bewildered, violated and punished', processed by experts, without discussion, in rooms where 'powerful people are going to do horrible things to you'. May (1992) takes up the theme of the power relationship between the recipient of care and the professional providing that care through the professional practice of surveillance and objectification—i.e. treating the patient as a 'thing' to be processed rather than a human with basic needs to be cared for. Through such practices, the subjective experience becomes irrelevant to the overriding importance of the workings of the woman's uterus and body, which can be fixed when things go wrong (Rothman 1982).

Mastery, then, is a question of the woman feeling that she is 'really giving birth in an active sense to her own child' (Oakley 1983). Being enabled to use coping skills and to influence the decision-making processes means that women are not surrendering themselves to the professionals' control—they themselves are powerful. The idea of power is an important one to consider, because we as midwives are perceived as holding the knowledge base through our education and thus, it may be argued, we dominate the

women we care for by disabling their own active participation in their birth. Mastery is about transforming the knowledge base by sharing it with women, involving them and enabling their own power. Consider the words of the following participant:

'I'd more or less done it on me own. I felt proud, very proud and me boyfriend were proud. I liked to know what it felt like, just felt it and coped. They're [the midwives] helping you, you feel as though you want to do it.'

For the women in this study, the attending midwife either enabled or disabled their sense of mastery. When it came to having respect for choice, allowing control of self and of the decision-making processes, and sharing the professional knowledge base, midwives appeared to fall into two distinct categories. Some women perceived that the midwife 'commanded her will' (Foucault 1976), governing the woman through the use of the professional gaze, thereby disabling the sense of mastery. These women were humiliated and assumed the role of the compliant patient (Arney & Neil 1982):

'It was the lack of control, feeling as though I wasn't in control, I wasn't as involved as I expected to be. She [the midwife] controlled the birth totally. I wasn't working with her. I felt as though I'd had my body taken over by someone else, that I would have to do as I was told. I remember fighting her 'cos I wanted to be sat up and she wouldn't let me. I was being pushed back down.'

'It was more of a midwife controlled birth. I felt as though I was up there somewhere out of control, not really participating.'

'They put me on a monitor. I wish I could have got up more. All I wanted to do was get up, walk about. But you can't, can you?'

'There was no discussion about breaking my waters and the hormone drip. I had no control over what was going on. It would have been nice for somebody to sit down and said, "Well this is what's going to happen, these are the options"—just to know what's going on.'

Thus we have those midwives who use their knowledge benevolently in order to facilitate the woman's own power in terms of her body and her self-knowledge, to enable the woman to make her birth her own. Unfortunately, some women were dominated because their midwife took on the role of an objective onlooker rather than one of a carer offering patience, support and comfort.

Subjective and objective: the mind and body experience fragmentation

Riley (1977) and Oakley (1977) write of the 'wholeness' of the birth experience and the division of the mind and body through pain parallels with the objective and subjective within midwifery care. The objective is said to be what is medically and physically done to the woman, the measurement of her physiology, while the subjective is what is felt or experienced by her. By implication, if we give care within the prevailing medical model, with its emphasis on treating the pregnant body as one that is ill and whose parts are capable of being fixed, the division between objective and subjective is clear: the subjective, unlike the objective, cannot be measured and is therefore of less concern, marginal to the real work of the woman's uterus which is to expel the baby (Martin 1989).

The physiological workings cause the pain of labour, but physiology and the concept of self, that is the mental, emotional and social needs, cannot be separated, as the model of medical dominance would have us believe. An integrated approach is required, so that care meets the woman's needs for both physical and emotional comfort during childbirth.

Martin's (1989) study reflects the split between the mind and the body, whereby women describe a sense of being divided from their body as a result of scientific, objective treatment at the expense of their concept of self. The feeling of not being in control of their bodily pain was also expressed to me by the women in this study, and this feeling of fragmentation was enhanced either through the drugs they were given or through analgesia being insufficient or inappropriate to need. This in turn meant that birth was no longer an event that they could actively experience (Martin 1989). The women described a feeling of being detached from their bodies through pain; all expressed their need to be in control of both their minds and their bodies. In view of this interaction between mind and body, it is probably ill-conceived to attempt to isolate physical care from emotional support. The following are direct quotes of participants describing their sensations:

'I felt a lot easier then [after epidural], I started talking then. I felt better, clear head. I weren't stressed out or anything. I were alright. I'd thought in me mind, that pain, that pain were worse than owt I'd ever ... It's like a stabbing, really grinding at you.'

'Contractions came thick and fast. I was shouting, "Don't have a baby, it's agony! I don't want any more pain, torture, constant torture." I cried like a high pitched scream, a strange cry. My mind looking at husband trying to be calmer, but after a while, I just went back again and I just felt out of control again. I thought rational things during being irrational. I got lost in it.'

'I didn't realise the knockout effect it [pethidine] would have and I felt totally out of control and I missed a lot of what went on in my mind. I missed the most important part at the end and I felt that I'd had my body taken over. I wanted to be more aware, I didn't realise the head was halfway out.'

'I was in that much pain, couldn't coordinate gas mask on me face, I couldn't focus. You're like on another planet, you're still there but it feels like you're on another planet. It's weird, you just go numb. It takes your mind off the pain. The pain was overwhelming, overwhelming.'

The need for interaction between woman and midwife was paramount: being with and being there; being valued as an individual

It became apparent through the women's testimonies that some midwives focused on the interpersonal process and were able to use the fact of being there, as people, in a therapeutic way (Munhall & Oiler 1986). In these cases, the woman felt that the midwife was trying to create an authentic personal relationship, trying to know her personally and subjectively rather than objectifying her as something to be processed quickly through the system: this was 'being there and being with' women. Carper (1978) helps us to understand the way in which some practitioners instinctively know how to create the opportunity for another person's growth and development— in this case the transformation of woman to mother through being connected with women during caring interactions.

The participants themselves described this kind of beneficial care from midwives who knew how to be with women:

'They were there when you needed them and not there when you didn't need them. It amazed me how they knew when to be there and when not to be. Very supportive, I could turn to them. I was really impressed, they're there for you all the way. She stood there about 10 minutes and talked me through it. She was so perceptive, she really picked up on it. She got me in the bath and it was like a new beginning.' (This woman had had a long and arduous first stage of labour and a new midwife had brought her new hope.)

'Patience, patience, coax you, praise you, they're helping you. The midwife helped me along with the breathing, a constant presence.'

'By the way she talked, she made me feel comfortable, explaining. I felt better even though I did have pain. She did care, the one that stopped with me most of the time, she were there to hold me hand, she stayed with me. I liked the comfort when she held me hand.'

The above women were enabled, they were safe and strong, they perceived their own control. And yet other women, through careless care, were rendered vulnerable, at the weak end of a power situation; they were dominated by the midwife, within the institution, their control of their bodies shifting, their self-esteem lost; they were no longer of value as their expressed needs were neither believed nor met. They succumbed to the clinical gaze (Foucault 1976) whereby humiliation plus control means a compliant and accepting patient, the woman being disabled and unable to accept responsibility for herself in making the transition to mother as a result of her accepting patienthood and professional domination.

'She said, "It's only Braxton Hicks"—she was demeaning my ability to tell how I felt. I thought, "You don't know how I feel." It was the way she dismissed them and I felt that she didn't believe what I was saying. I didn't feel as though I'd been asked anything. Nobody actually asked me what position I'd thought of for the birth. She took over and did her job.'

'I didn't feel as though I bonded with the midwife, I needed gentle persuasion, sympathy. I need the soft touch. I was always aware of her facial expression, I can't remember her smiling at me. Her presence was professionally helpful but there was no support emotionally. I wanted somebody to hold my hand, perhaps put their arm around me instead of being spoken to as though I was doing wrong. She kept saying, "Pull yourself together, you've got to pull yourself together." I just felt that I didn't get adequate pain relief really, unfortunately the epidural didn't work. I was conscious that I had to be good for her all the time. She was very professional and distant. I remember her going out and thinking, "Well I haven't formed a relationship with you." I think I'll be scared for the next time.'

I have included this detailed example of a woman's feelings as it highlights a few issues relating to the midwife 'being with'; to professional control through demeaning another; to pain relief; and to the need for connections between the woman and the midwife. Childbirth is a common yet unique experience for the individual woman,

and various authors have written of the feelings of being out of control through pain and lack of information as direct reinforcers of not being able to cope or perform adequately during birth (Richards 1982, Ong 1983, Kirkham 1989).

At the heart of this discussion is the need for real communication between women and midwives, alongside the existence of a social relationship rather than a one-off meeting between two strangers, one (the woman) being more vulnerable than the other (the midwife) because of pain and a less 'expert' knowledge base. In turn, midwives can share their knowledge in an attempt to place the women at the centre of the action, and to enable them to feel their own sense of power. In this respect, Kelpin (1984) urges fellow women to 'accept and take hold of power, to literally and figuratively "stand up" and actively birth our own children rather than be delivered of our children'.

The significance of the sensations of birth makes the wholeness of the experience

The women spoke spontaneously of the uniqueness of the sensations of the baby moving through their pelvis towards birth and each woman viewed it as a positive experience. Their testimonies speak for themselves:

'The best were seeing her! And you can feel her as well, feel her head. "Oh gosh, it's nearly here!" Oh, it were brilliant!'

'I could feel, they weren't strong but I could feel them, so I knew. "Really push down, really push down!" So I gave it a right good push and then it were all over! And I looked, but I liked it really, I liked it! It just all seemed to get pushed away— she were there and it were alright!'

'I pushed and she just came out. I just felt her, whole of her, the whole thing. Very quick, you've got to feel something.'

'I started pushing, I could feel it moving down, pains were really strong. I were just overwhelmed, I just bent over and had a look at her—it were lovely!'

'I wanted to feel the head but I didn't actually feel the head going down. Nobody said—so sad really. The thing I missed most was not touching her head. I wanted her to be delivered onto my tummy but nobody asked me about that.'

'When she was being born, I remember her telling me to push, now I didn't actually realise that the head was halfway out. I just remember thinking I wasn't happy with where I wanted to be.'

'You go through this experience and at the end of it there's this wonderful thing, this baby! You need to know that you've done a good job really!'

The women's lived experience of care by midwives

In order to pull together the analysis of the women's lived experiences, this full description acts as a summary of all events:

• The sense of having mastery of their birth was an essential component for this group of women and this was enhanced by midwives who had respect for the woman's need for choice, and for control of herself and her own decision-making processes. When these needs were met, the women had the sense of being valued as individuals and their coping abilities were enabled. A dehumanised picture of care was apparent when these needs were not appreciated by the midwife and therefore not met; in these cases, the women appeared to spiral into a situation of domination and pain from which they could not escape.

• Those midwives who were perceived as using themselves in a therapeutic way during their relationship with the women gave beneficial care. The nature of this behaviour related to being with the women and offering patience, support and comfort, and being there for them when needed, thus enabling them through their pain and birth experience.

• Those women whose self-esteem needs were met were able to feel powerful within their pain of labour, as their minds and bodies were supported emotionally and physically by the midwife through the process of working towards the birth. Sadly, not all women received such care; they became objects of the organisation, a case to be processed by midwives who were seemingly unable to develop useful interpersonal relationships of empathy and understanding.

DISCUSSION AND REFLECTIONS

The birth attendant for the majority of women in Britain today is a midwife who is present to give support, advice and comfort, and to make available a range of midwifery skills as and when

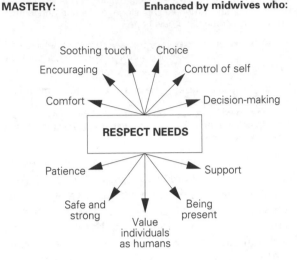

Figure 7.1   A model for care by midwives.

these might be required by the women in her care (Richards 1982; see also Fig. 7.1). In order that a helping relationship might be developed, interaction between the woman and the midwife is paramount, with the midwife responding appropriately to the woman's stated needs using her repertoire of skills to pick up on the woman's verbal and non-verbal cues, and creating a climate of openness and trust whereby both woman and midwife can grow and develop (Mayeroff 1971, Rogers 1983) through mutual respect of each other's life and learning.

It is not what the midwife *does* physically to the woman in her care during childbirth; more importantly, it is what the midwife *is* when undertaking care. This can be defined, taking heed of the women in this study, as being present both physically and mentally for women; and not demeaning the woman's need for help, however that may be expressed.

The spontaneous mentions of the mind/body or subject/object view of themselves during labour was a revelation to me as a practising midwife who is also a mother, and the women's testimonies enabled my own birth recollections whereby one is rational in thought yet one's body is controlled by its physical forces. To be attended by a midwife who herself is controlling through objectification of one's body and who lacks the skills of nurture and comfort could indeed, as Hunt & Symonds (1995) suggest, marginalise the lived experience of a fulfilling birth.

We now have access to a wealth of literature to support the perceived 'soft' concepts of caring (Benner & Wrubel 1989, Forrest 1989). The value of such caring attributes are essential to the recipients, and yet within midwifery practice great emphasis is still placed upon the role of technologist—e.g. observing the monitor and applying the scalp electrode—rather than the emotional effort of being with women. Both Kirkham (1989) and Hunt & Symonds (1995), in their qualitative studies of the labour ward, expressed this view of midwives entrenched within a medical model, with tasks and roles delegated by medical domination appearing to be viewed as more important than a nurturing, supportive role, which often goes on behind closed doors and which is implicitly less valued than the end result: a delivery.

The nature of this study allowed a small group of women to be subjective about their birth experience. They were literally enabled to 'debrief' and it was remarkable how eager the women were to talk it through, almost to relive it. As one woman stated: 'It's nice to talk through the whole thing from beginning to end—just to talk it out makes you feel so much better.'

There appeared to be a sense of release and this raises the question of whether opportunities should be created to enable women to 'talk themselves out' (Bogdan & Taylor 1984) in the busy environment of postnatal wards where privacy needs are at a premium and time is of the essence.

It is not intended that the sample size of seven women should offer the ability to generalise to other situations, as it was chosen for convenience in an attempt to organise the large amount of qualitative data. However, subjective accounts of care received do have a purpose for health care professionals who may feel puzzled at women's desires to make meaningful choices and decisions about their care and progress during childbirth, which is often viewed as fighting against the prevailing obstetric viewpoint of medical dominance.

The alternative model of 'mastery' (see Fig. 7.2), whereby women and midwives share the planning

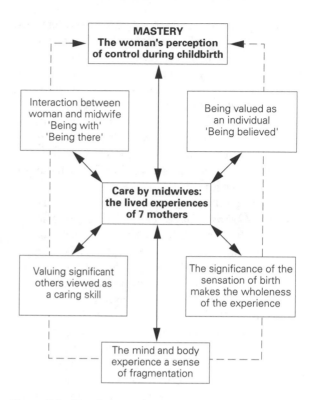

Figure 7.2 Results.

of care based on the concepts of control of decision-making, taking responsibility for choices made, and the encouragement of self-esteem, is at the furthest extreme from medicalised care and means working in alliance with women. Such care strategies form the basis of *Changing Childbirth* (Department of Health 1993), and if midwifery is to be woman-centred then women's experiential views of childbirth deserve to be heard in order that we may create challenges to existing ideologies of care.

REFLECTIONS OF MY PRACTICE RELATED TO THE RESEARCH

By using a phenomenological approach to interviewing and analysis of the data, one aims to facilitate the woman's telling of her interpretation of her experiences. It means asking focusing but not leading questions and listening carefully with concentration (Harvey 1993). During the earliest interviews this focusing did not always occur, as my inexperience led me to ask directive questions, controlling by putting my point of view as a midwife rather than being receptive. This situation arose particularly when a woman revealed her pain at being demeaned by the midwife attending her: 'I just felt as though I lost participation. I was just a body to be y' know delivered. I just got the idea that it had become a job to them.'

My reaction was of deep sorrow for this woman and I became aware that I was trying to 'put things right' for her, consequently talking too much, controlling the flow of conversation. It was at this stage that I realised that a debriefing session after the interviews was essential to provide emotional support after difficult self-disclosure (May 1991). I was constantly reminded of the power issues within the relationship between myself and the women as they were captives within the institution of which I was a part, and, as the stories unfolded, the recurrent theme of control of women by others was central. I took the view that, through enabling the women to tell their stories with freedom to express and explore their present and future needs, the control of the data was theirs and that they had accepted the opportunity to value and share their unique experiences.

Kirkham (1994) comments on the usefulness of the telling of stories by mothers and midwives as a method of research but more importantly as a method of caring, and we as midwives can utilise such strategies to enhance our skills. The analysis of the data provided me with the ideal opportunity to reflect on what the women were saying about midwifery care, how they were striving to understand what had happened to them, how they could integrate this with the rest of their life and how I, as a practitioner, could benefit from the knowledge they offered me.

I came to realise that my own care giving was in a transitional phase, from the strong skills-based approach applied to women's needs to a more receptive approach based on their experiences to which I could add my insight, if required, as a midwife with certain knowledge and skills to offer. This is a crucial difference to be aware of, if midwives are to offer care based upon women's expressed needs rather than processing

them through what Hunt & Symonds (1995) call the assembly line 'factory production process'.

Having such a reflective approach, which consists of being present for a woman and listening to her needs as an individual, providing comfort and trust, is indeed emotionally and physically draining and requires more than the manual dexterity of delivering the baby. It means that we must relate to women, that is 'being for' each other, in such a way that both people involved in the caring relationship feel that the relationship is enhanced (Tschudin 1987). It also means spending time with women, facilitating a supportive network of colleagues and having managers who view such in-depth working patterns as essential and who have a philosophy of care which promotes women's needs above professional power needs. Maybe this is too idealistic for hard-pressed midwives who themselves are often oppressed by both their management and medical structures.

SUMMARY

As this study shows, many women still have starkly different experiences of childbirth, and these differences often relate to how 'in control' of the situation they felt they were. In turn, this feeling of being in control or out of control seems to have been exacerbated one way or the other by the way in which the attending midwife approached the process of giving birth. It is clear, therefore, that some concerted effort is required on the part of all midwives to ensure a consistent approach which moves away from the medicalised view of childbirth that has been in the ascendancy in recent decades.

Changing Childbirth (Department of Health 1993) has provided midwives with an opportunity to create this kind of change, if they have the energy and commitment for it. If we do not take up this challenge then I suggest that, as this research shows, some women will continue to receive 'care' which erodes their capacity to cope, and erodes their control of their own minds, bodies and pain—i.e. care which, as Foucault (1976) suggests, controls by its professional knowledge base of power, through objectifying women by doing things to them rather than nurturing them by sharing the caring knowledge to enable their empowerment.

REFERENCES

Arney W, Neil J 1982 The location of pain in childbirth: natural childbirth and the transformation of obstetrics. Sociology of Health and Illness 4: 1

Benner P, Wrubel J 1989 The primacy of caring. Addison Wesley, New York

Bogdan R, Taylor S J 1984 Introduction to qualitative research methods. Wiley, New York

Carper B A 1978 Fundamental patterns of knowing in nursing. Advances in Nursing Science 1 (1): 13–23

Colaizzi P 1978 Psychological research as the phenomenologist views it. In: Valle E, King M (eds) Existential phenomenological alternatives for psychology. Oxford University Press, New York

Darbyshire P 1994 Understanding caring through arts and humanities : a medical/nursing humanities approach to promoting alternative experiences of thinking and learning. Journal of Advanced Nursing 19 (5): 856

Department of Health 1993 Changing childbirth. HMSO, London

Forrest D 1989 The experience of caring. Journal of Advanced Nursing 14: 815–823

Foucault M 1976 The birth of the clinic. Tavistock, London

Graham H 1983 Caring: a labour of love. In: Finch J, Groves D (eds) A labour of love. Women work and caring. Routledge Kegan, London

Harvey S 1993 The genesis of a phenomenological approach to advanced nursing practice. Journal of Advanced Nursing 18: 526–530

Harwood J 1988 Home comforts. Midwives Chronicle: Sept, 266–268

Hunt S, Symonds A 1995 The social meaning of midwifery. Macmillan, London

Kelpin V 1984 Birthing pain. Phenomenology and Pedagogy 2 (2): 178–187

Kirkham M 1986 A feminist perspective in midwifery. In: Webb C (ed) Feminist practice in women's health care. John Wiley, Chichester

Kirkham M 1989 Midwives and information giving in labour. In: Robinson S, Thomson A (eds) Midwives, research and childbirth, vol 1. Chapman and Hall, London

Kirkham M 1994 Using research skills in midwifery practice. British Journal of Midwifery 2 (8): 390–392

Martin E 1989 The woman in the body. Oxford University Press, London

May C 1992 Individual care? Power and subjectivity in therapeutic relationships. Sociology 26 (4): 589–602

May K 1991 Interviewing. In: Morse J (ed) Qualitative nursing research. Sage, California

Mayeroff M 1971 On caring. Harper Row, London

Munhall P, Oiler C 1986 Nursing research. A qualitative perspective. Appleton Century Croft, Connecticut

Murphy-Black T 1995 Issues in midwifery. Churchill Livingstone, London

Oakley A 1977 Cross cultural practices. In: Chard T, Richards M (eds) Benefits and hazards of the new obstetrics. Heinemann, London

Oakley A 1983 Social consequences of obstetric technology: the importance of measuring soft outcomes. Birth 10 (2): 106

Omery A 1983 Phenomenology, a method for nursing research. Advances in Nursing Science 5(2): 49–63

Ong B N 1983 Our motherhood. Women's accounts of pregnancy, childbirth and health encounters. Family Service Units, London

Raphael-Leff J 1990 Psychological processes of childbearing. Chapman and Hall, London

Richards M P M 1982 The trouble with choice in childbirth. Birth 9 (4): 253–261

Riley E 1977 What do women want? The question of choice in the conduct of labour. In: Chard T, Richards M (eds) Benefits and hazards of the new obstetrics. Heinemann, London

Rogers C 1983 Freedom to learn for the 80's. Bell and Howell Co, USA

Rothman B 1982 In labour: women and power in the birthplace. Norton and Co, New York

Stanley L 1991 Feminist praxis. Routledge, London

Tschudin V 1987 Counselling skills for nurses. Balliere Tindall, London

8

Complementary medicine for pain control in labour

Sue Moore and Miranda Holden

LEARNING OUTCOMES

At the end of this chapter the reader will have

- **an introduction to the principles of complementary therapies**

- **identified the professional responsibilities of the midwife in relation to the training and use of complementary therapies and Statutory requirements**

- **an introduction to some of the main therapies which are effective in reducing or relieving pain in labour: massage, aromatherapy, homeopathy, acupuncture, reflexology, hypnotherapy and self-hypnosis, yoga, meditation and therapeutic breathwork, herbalism and naturopathy**

- **identified sources for further information and general enquires relating to complementary therapies.**

Over the past 15 years the field of complementary therapies has become tremendously popular with the general public, as many people are seeking a more holistic approach to health care. It has also gained a new-found credibility amongst the medical profession, as researchers begin to gather new evidence to validate some of the oldest healing methods known to humans.

Complementary medicine is an umbrella term for a variety of healing arts. Although unique in their application, most therapies share similar principles, aiming to treat the whole person— body, mind and spirit—believing that an imbalance in one area of life will create an effect in another. This principle is most easily demonstrated by the tangible results that stress can have on our physical body, such as contributing to stomach ulcers, hypertension and irritable bowel syndrome, and the relationship between the things we eat and our mood.

Complementary therapies offer a less invasive form of health care than many forms of traditional medicine and aim to treat the cause of imbalance rather than suppressing symptoms. Complementary medicine supports the client in making the necessary changes to their lifestyle in order to eliminate the causes of the imbalance, be that emotional, environmental or physical. Proponents of complementary medicine also uphold the belief that prevention is better than cure, and support people in taking responsibility for improving and maintaining their health as an ongoing commitment, thereby helping to prevent or control common degenerative conditions such as arthritis, cancer and heart disease. This holistic approach will often help expectant mothers to feel empowered. In addition, some of the complementary approaches outlined in this chapter are believed to help reduce the incidence of complications and unnecessary trauma for mother and baby.

There are many different complementary therapies available, offering powerful, safe, yet gentle options for pain management during labour. Although developments in modern medicine have greatly increased the safety of childbirth for mother and baby, it is important to remember that the process of pregnancy and birth is not an illness, but one of nature's true miracles! Natural therapies have much to offer the pregnant woman, however, like orthodox medicine, they too have their limitations. Most natural therapists are keen to see a merging of the two different schools of medicine to provide the most comprehensive and appropriate form of health care to every person. This chapter will outline the major natural therapies available, and their value and application in minimising pain during labour.

COMPLEMENTARY THERAPY AND MIDWIFERY PRACTICE

Midwives have a professional responsibility and are accountable for all areas of their practice. The *Midwives' Rules* (UKCC 1993) and *The Midwife's Code of Practice* (1994) are regulated, published and made available to every registered midwife by the United Kingdom Central Council for Nurses, Midwives and Health Visitors (UKCC). As stated in the *Code of Practice*:

… each midwife as a practitioner is responsible for her own practice in whatever environment she practices. The standard of practice in the delivery of care shall be that which is acceptable in the context of current knowledge and clinical developments. In all circumstances the safety and welfare of the mother and her baby must be of primary importance.

Midwives have a particular responsibility for the administration of medicines and other forms of pain relief (UKCC 1993, Rule 41). In relation to Rule 40 (responsibilities and sphere of practice), the UKCC (1994) state:

Other developments in midwifery and obstetric practice may also require new skills, but these skills do not necessarily become an integral part of the role of all midwives. In such circumstances each employing authority should have locally agreed policies which observe the Council's requirements and National Board advice and guidance. You should familiarise yourself with the policies of any authority in which you may practice.

Midwives are responsible for maintaining and developing their professional competence and skills in all aspects of practice, which will include the use of complementary therapies. It is therefore implicit that every midwife should ensure that she is fully cognisant with the particular therapy she may be planning to use and that she has been adequately trained in its use. She also has a responsibility to consult with her supervisor of midwives regarding preparation and experience when considering acquiring new skills (UKCC 1994).

The *Midwife's Code of Practice* provides specific standards for the administration of homeopathic or herbal substances and for the use of complementary and alternative therapies, as do the

Standards for the administration of medicines (UKCC 1992). Midwives should always refer to these standards before considering the use of such therapies. Naturally, midwives also have to consider the woman's choice in what she may want to use for relief of pain in labour. *Changing Childbirth* (Department of Health 1993) sets the agenda for action and change which is necessary for achieving the overall aim of woman-centred care:

The woman should feel secure in the knowledge that she can make her choice after full discussion of all the issues with the professionals involved in her care. She should feel confident that these professionals will respect her right to choose her care on that basis, and ensure that the services provided are of the best quality possible.

THERAPEUTIC MASSAGE

The use of pressure and massage to encourage relaxation and release tension is one of the oldest, simplest and most immediate healing tools available to the midwife. A knowledge of anatomy and physiology is essential, as is practical training of the various strokes, but nothing could be more important to a woman in labour than a midwife who has built a trusting rapport with the mother. Some mothers seek help from professional massage therapists to ease back pain and encourage relaxation during pregnancy, and subsequently may bring their massage therapist with them into the labour ward. This usually works well, as the therapist has already built up a trusting relationship with the mother and can therefore work with the midwife to support the woman and help to relieve her pain.

It is a natural, intuitive response for many midwives to massage the woman in labour. Midwives should feel encouraged to trust their intuition and gain confidence in a natural form of therapy and pain relief. Many midwives routinely use gentle back massage as part of their practice. Although there are many techniques for massage, most women will say when they do not want to be touched or if the form of massage is not to their liking.

Most massage therapists like to give a full body massage once labour has begun, and then to work deeply over the lower back, and legs in a downward and outward motion when contractions are more established. Massage during labour is highly personal. Some women find that massage during the contractions helps to relieve and 'spread' the pain, while others prefer to be left alone and then massaged after each major contraction to relax and soothe tired muscles. Massage is very helpful at decreasing the intensity of the pain; by reducing tension, pain becomes less localised and often easier to cope with. It is important to be flexible and to communicate with the woman as to her particular preferences.

All of the massage strokes should be focused on spreading and dissipating tension. It is often recommended that massage should be performed in a downward and outward fan-like motion, applying pressure with the thumbs. It is general practice by some therapists not to massage the abdomen of pregnant women, but to focus on the lower back, hips and legs. However, some midwives trained in aromatherapy use a gentle massage with oils over the abdomen. This is found to be relaxing and is enjoyed by the women on whom it is performed. Often the mother's shoulders, neck and jaw will be tense, and massaging these areas will help her to relax and breathe more evenly. If there is trembling in the legs, massaging downwards with strong pressure from the hips to the feet has been reported to be very effective.

It can be extremely beneficial for the woman's partner to learn massage skills well before the birth, as many mothers may feel most comfortable being massaged during labour by someone with whom they have a deep bond. For some women, particularly if opting for a natural birth, having either a massage therapist or the midwife working 'deeply' on the spine and hips from behind works better, with their partner free to offer emotional support and encouragement.

Many midwives are deepening their understanding of, and skill at carrying out, massage techniques. There are many courses offering training in massage and aromatherapy, as well as other complementary therapies. It is important that midwives ensure that the course they are undertaking is suitable for use in professional practice. Details of useful contacts for advice can be found at the end of this chapter.

AROMATHERAPY

Aromatherapy is the art of using the concentrated oils from plants and flowers which are believed to have specific healing and 'balancing' properties on the mind and body. The oils are usually diluted with a carrier oil and massaged onto the skin, diluted in a bath, or inhaled through the use of an oil burner.

The essential oils are extracts of plants which have various therapeutic properties. The oils are highly concentrated and contain many chemical components. Although these oils have an effective therapeutic effect, there are potential adverse effects, of which every aromatherapist will be aware. Aromatherapists use several different techniques for blending the oils. The chemical constituents of the oils stimulate the body to balance itself, and appear to help women cope with the pain and the process of labour on a physical level as well as an emotional level. The essential oils are blended with a base oil such as sweet almond or sesame seed oil. Essential oils are stored in dark brown bottles, but occasionally blue bottles are used. Many oils which are available on the market are not pure oils but are of a much poorer quality, and are often sold in clear bottles. Essential oils are fairly expensive because of the very laborious process of extracting the oils from the plants. Some, such as sandalwood, are very expensive.

It is standard practice for aromatherapists to ask their client to smell the oils that are indicated for use before applying them. Our sense of smell is highly personal, and will evoke memories and feelings unique to every individual. Aromatherapy is believed to work primarily through the limbic system, assisting in the relaxation and uplifting of mental and emotional states, which then exerts an effect on the body. It is known that this part of the nervous system is implicated in emotional and memory processes within the brain and it is therefore believed to be this area which is activated by aromatherapy. It is

vital that the oils used are agreeable to the mother's sense of smell, as it is unlikely that oils to which the person has an aversion will exert a therapeutic effect. Most people will intuitively select oils that will be most helpful to them at the time. Always waft the oils under the mother's nose to check her emotional response. Pregnant women appear to have a particularly sensitive sense of smell; aromatherapy mixtures should therefore not be too concentrated.

Aromatherapy in conjunction with massage is perhaps one complementary therapy for which training is now accessible to many midwives as courses are being presented nation-wide in colleges of higher education, and some universities are even running degree programmes. The following section will present the experience of one midwife, Dee Cooper, who practises in a large maternity hospital in a multicultural, inner city area. Dee is now offering her skills in aromatherapy to the women who present in pregnancy and labour, as well as providing colleagues with a method of unwinding at times of stress. Midwives are committed to giving women attending the unit choices for labour, particularly regarding methods of pain relief. Dee presents some of the issues which were raised in her aromatherapy training and also presents some case studies. It is anticipated that the experience of these women in labour will encourage readers to discuss the issues, reflect on practice and participate in setting up further research into the effectiveness of complementary therapies in labour.

Experiences of Dee Cooper, midwife

'Throughout my training as an aromatherapist, much emphasis was placed on the environment, that is the surroundings, as well as the type of relationship built up with the individual within the consultation process. The client's medical, physical and social history, her lifestyle, including amount of exercise, diet, drinking habits and relaxation, are routinely discussed. Many conditions are stress-related and the consultation can give the therapist an insight into any problems the client may have.

'The skills gained by a midwife in assessing a woman's physical and psychological needs, as well as the natural process of building a relationship, help in reducing the time that many aromatherapists might need for a normal consultation. A midwife also has a detailed knowledge of the woman's physical and medical history throughout pregnancy. The consultation is therefore part of the welcoming and admitting process, especially in labour, helping to put the woman and her birth partner(s) at ease. As the recommendations of *Changing Childbirth* are implemented, and women are cared for by smaller numbers of midwives, it is anticipated that this aspect of care will become even more apparent.

'The case studies in Boxes 8.1–8.3 are examples of women who have found aromatherapy and massage effective at varying stages of their labours. (The names are fictitious to protect confidentiality). It is recognised that ideally the woman

---

Box 8.1 Case study: Sharon

Sharon, 20 years of age and expecting her first baby, had presented several times throughout her pregnancy with urinary tract infections (UTIs), understandably believing she was in labour on some of these occasions. She had been admitted to hospital twice, and had met the midwives and familiarised herself with the labour ward. She also got to know the midwife who would eventually care for her in labour. Sharon's mother was planning to be with her throughout labour. When Sharon was eventually admitted in early labour, she was welcomed and admitted by a midwife whom she knew. Although in very early labour, she chose to stay in the hospital rather than spend a little more time at home. Sharon eventually started to use TENS (transcutaneous electrical nerve stimulation), and had an injection of pethidine. At that time her contractions were still irregular and cervical dilation was minimal. She then requested an epidural; unfortunately it was not effective.

Several hours later, Sharon was becoming extremely distressed. She had an epidural catheter *in situ* which was serving no purpose, an intravenous infusion in progress, and was attached to a fetal monitor. Initially the midwife needed to establish a close rapport with Sharon, and with lots of encouragement (including a comforting cuddle) was eventually able to build up trust and reassure her that she was going to get through her labour. Next, the epidural catheter and intravenous infusion were removed. Sharon became calmer immediately and she chose to mobilise, adopting various positions including squatting and 'all fours'. Intermittent auscultation was performed to monitor fetal well-being, as the baby was coping well with labour.

Four drops of essential oils of lavender (*Lavendula augustifolia*), and 4 drops of German chamomile (*Matricaria recutica*) were mixed in a 25 ml base of sweet almond oil and then used to massage Sharon's back. Sharon quickly gained full control of the situation, and began intermittent pushing with contractions. She began to take control of her body, pushing when she felt she wanted to. She was now calm and adopted an 'all-fours' position to give birth, now in complete control although verbalising that 'she couldn't do it'. Sharon gave birth to a baby boy with her partner and her mother present, giving support. The third stage was uneventful and she had an intact perineum. Sharon has since had her second baby and spent much of that labour in a bath fragranced with chamomile and lavender. She gave birth to a baby girl, again in the 'all-fours' position, and choosing back massage. Chamomile and lavender have a relaxing and calming effect and therefore would appear to have had a good therapeutic effect for this mother.

Box 8.2 Case study: Shamim

Shamim was expecting her first baby, and did not speak or understand English. Her birth partners were her mother-in-law and her aunt, who both acted as interpreters. Shamim was in established labour and lay on the bed in obvious pain. With the help of her birth partners it was suggested to Shamim that she may feel less pain if she was in a more upright position. Shamim tried this and with the support of her birth partners found it helpful to walk about. Her supporters were very encouraging, massaging her back and making 'kneading' movements to her hips. The possible advantage of introducing essential oils was discussed and Shamim thought this may be helpful with the massage. Ylang ylang (*Cananga odorata*), chamomile (*Matricaria recutica*) and clary sage (*Salvia sclarea*) in a ratio of 3 + 3 + 2 drops, were mixed with a 25 ml sweet almond oil base, for Shamim's massage.

As the aroma filled the room, the aunt informed me that this was good, it was helping Shamim and it was just like it would be in her own country. The three of them were a team, and Shamim progressed in labour, needing no other pain relief.

Box 8.3 Case study: Susan

Susan (expecting her first baby) was admitted from the antenatal ward to delivery suite in established labour (cervix 8 cm dilated) and using TENS. She had been able to maintain a good breathing pattern during contractions, appeared to be in control but now felt in need of additional pain relief. She appeared happy and relaxed and was accompanied by her husband Andy. Susan wished to maintain an upright position and so she sat in a rocking chair supported by pillows. She began to use Entonox during contractions. Susan and Andy had both attended parentcraft classes and had brought their own essential oils with them to use during labour. After a brief demonstration from the midwife, Andy began to massage Susan's neck and shoulders which she found very relaxing, and it also allowed Andy to become involved in the labour. As her labour progressed she stood and leaned on the bed, but as she began to feel more tired she moved onto the bed, on all fours, resting the top half of her body on a bean bag and pillows. In this position she was able to cope with the pain, and remained in control. Andy was able to massage Susan's lower back and sacral area and buttocks with geranium oil and this helped to facilitate a relaxed state as she approached transition. At this point Susan asked for the TENS to be removed so that Andy could continue with the massage effectively. To help with transition she relaxed in a warm bath with chamomile and lavender oil. Thirty minutes later, Susan was experiencing a strong urge to push and she then moved to a birthing stool. With Andy sitting beside her for support, she was able to maintain eye contact with her birth attendants, and using a mirror they were both able to view the baby's head as it advanced. Susan instinctively made maternal effort as her body dictated, adjusting her breathing pattern in response. As their baby daughter was born they were able to experience the exhilaration of the first eye contact with their infant as Susan cradled the baby in her arms and Andy leaned forward to cut the umbilical cord.

will have met her midwife and discussed the use of aromatherapy well before labour. Some of these cases are the exceptions.

'As yet there is very little research to validate the effectiveness of aromatherapy alone when used in labour. Like many other aspects relating to care in labour, there are so many other influencing variables, not least of all the subjectivity of pain perception. It is therefore not appropriate to administer a basic mix of essential oils for everyone, as when prescribing a dose of paracetamol.

'The cases have mainly involved active birth, however essential oils have a place in many other situations, especially in the labour ward. It can be used in the waiting area to relax anxious visitors and waiting relatives. When a woman has an epidural *in situ*, aromatherapy may still be used. I have found that massaging her hands can be very helpful. Women who have labour induced have responded well to a gentle abdominal massage of geranium, lavender and clary sage with one drop of cinnamon. Midwives are often confronted by women who hyperventilate in labour, a calming influence can be created by introducing frankincense to the basic mix.

'Finally, it is important to recognise that some people, including my midwifery colleagues, have an allergic type of sensitivity to essential oils. One of my colleagues is acutely sensitive to lavender, and only has to smell it to bring about a reaction. Midwives also become pregnant, and as advice to clients often includes avoiding certain therapies in the first trimester of pregnancy, midwives also need to be aware that administering aromatherapy is not really that different to receiving it, and therefore probably contraindicated.'

Application of aromatherapy oils

Never apply aromatherapy oils directly to the skin. Always mix with a carrier such as sweet almond oil, grapeseed oil or avocado oil, with a total of 2–3 drops of essential oil to every 5 ml of carrier oil (i.e. a 2–3% mix) for pregnancy and labour.

Massaging the mother in the initial stages of labour allows her to relax and focus her mind on the task ahead. A good combination of oils to use is lavender, chamomile, sandalwood/frankincense, and 2 drops of neroli, mixed with the carrier oil. These oils have the following qualities:

• Lavender is a very relaxing, balancing oil, with pain-relieving properties, and it blends well with many oils.

• Chamomile is very calming and relaxing, and is believed to be an anti-spasmodic and therefore good for pain relief. Chamomile oil can be obtained in German or Roman form. Moroccan is also available but may be less effective for labour.

• Frankincense is a relaxing oil which slows and deepens the breathing. This is excellent for asthmatics, if the mother is panicky or if there are complications, as it helps to dilate the bronchial vessels and ensure that the mother continues to breathe fully and deeply.

• Sandalwood is very similar to frankincense, with properties to aid relaxation and breathing, although it is slightly less overpowering and is fairly expensive to purchase. Use either frankincense or sandalwood, not both together.

• Neroli is a very uplifting oil which is thought to aid concentration and mental focus, and as such is necessary for the mother during childbirth. There is some evidence of its relaxing effect on patients undergoing intensive care (Stevenson 1992).

As labour progresses, other oils which may be helpful are:

• Geranium, a very 'balancing' oil. Its smell is heavy and yet sweet.

• Jasmine, a very uplifting oil which is believed to stimulate uterine contraction and therefore quicken the process of labour. This may be helpful to women with a history of difficult births. It is a very heady oil, believed to stimulate endorphins, and is therefore recommended towards the later stages of labour.

• Clary sage, a very heady oil which stimulates endorphins. It is therefore especially helpful for pain relief in the later stages of labour. It also has a relaxing effect and creates a sense of euphoria.

• Rose, with a very feminine smell, is calming and uplifting and therefore particularly suitable for labour. It is sometimes found to be most effective when mixed with geranium.

It is not recommended to use essential oils in water-birth pools, as there is a theoretical risk that direct contact with the oils could have a detrimental effect on the baby. Instead, massage the mother with the oils at the commencement of labour, and towel the excess off her body just before she begins to use the pool. By this time the oils will have already been absorbed through her skin and will be starting to take their effect, without any possible effect on the baby. However, a therapeutic effect can still be gained through the aroma circulating within the room, by using a burner.

Oils for inhalation

As labour progresses, it may be helpful to burn a combination of oils as follows: frankincense, to assist with relaxation and deep breathing; neroli for mental clarity and focus; and jasmine or clary sage to assist the stimulation of endorphins. Oil burners are now relatively easy to purchase. Many mothers find it helpful to have the oils dabbed onto a handkerchief to inhale, or to have the oils dabbed underneath their nose; some have even dabbed the oils on the mask or mouthpiece when inhaling Entonox.

HOMEOPATHY

Homeopathy is one of the safest and most popular natural therapies available. It works on the principle that 'like cures like', similar to the principle of vaccination. It was first used therapeutically by

Hahnemann in the early nineteenth century. A homeopath will use highly diluted extracts of disease states and plants which mirror the symptoms present in the patient. This seems to stimulate the healing process and bring the person back into balance. Homeopathy is equally helpful for mental and emotional symptoms as it is for physical problems.

Homeopathy is a very subtle medicine and the potencies vary in strength according to the amount of active substance used and how extensively it is prepared. The active ingredient is prepared in a solution and is potentised by a technique of shaking or tapping the mixture (Fig. 8.1). The more minute the active substance, the more it has been potentised, and therefore the stronger the effect of the medicine (probably one of the most controversial aspects of homeopathy). Homeopathic advice suggests that in pregnancy certain substances should be avoided as they can reduce the effectiveness of the remedies. These include caffeine (tea, coffee and cola drinks), codeine and strong flavours such as peppermint (often in toothpaste) (Webb 1992).

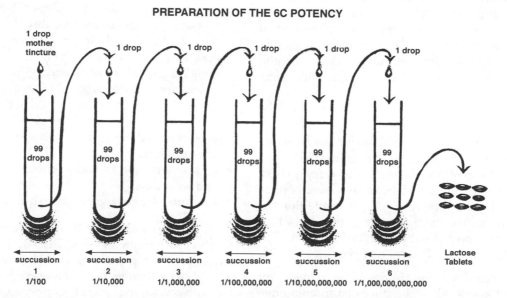

PREPARATION OF THE 6C POTENCY

Figure 8.1   Preparation of homeopathic potency 6C. Samuel Hahnemann, who first demonstrated the principle of homeopathy, used a method of dilution that involved a factor of one part in 100 parts. He also showed that at each stage of dilution vigorous shaking, known as succussion, conferred on this solution its homeopathic/therapeutic effect. (Reproduced with kind permission from Webb 1992.)

Dosages

The lowest dosage is 6 and is used for minor physical ailments. This is the strength generally available over the counter at health food stores and general pharmacies. A stronger dosage is 30 and this will normally be prescribed to help at the person's physical level. A dosage of 200 works on the physical and emotional level, often indicated where physical conditions are linked with a person's emotional state.

Stronger dosages used by experienced homeopaths include:

- 1 M is a strong dose working primarily on the mental level, also encompassing emotional and physical levels (this dosage has quite a powerful long-term effect)
- 10 M is one of the highest dosages available and it works on the spiritual, mental, emotional and physical levels.

These last two dosages are likely to have an effect for up to three months.

Every individual has inherited strengths and weaknesses—physical, mental and emotional—from their gene structure and their childhood environment, and will conform to one of several homeopathic constitutional types. Most homeopaths prefer to give ongoing constitutional treatment to strengthen a person's inherent weaknesses, thereby gradually strengthening their immune system over a period of time. Homeopathy, however, is also effective in bringing relief to acute symptoms, and has much to offer the pregnant woman.

Ideally, the mother would have been receiving constitutional treatment prior to conception, so as to be in the best possible health to carry a child, and she will continue to be treated by a homeopath during her pregnancy. Even where this has not been the case, there are several remedies which have been reported to be beneficial in labour. The three most commonly used remedies are:

- Arnica 30C—this is the main remedy for shock of any kind, and reduces pain, inflammation and bleeding, and promotes healing. It can be used at any point during and after labour for the simple physical and psychological strain.

- Hypericum 30C—again promotes healing and helps reduce tissue damage.
- Caulophyllum—this remedy is believed to strengthen contractions, and can greatly reduce the length and discomfort of labour. It is indicated if the contractions are weak, or if labour is not proceeding at a satisfactory rate and the mother is getting exhausted as a result. Some homeopaths believe this to be such a good remedy that every woman should have some before the birth; others argue that like any other remedy it should only be used if indicated. A history of difficult labours, or if the woman's own birth was difficult, is considered a reason for taking the remedy in advance. In this case the homeopath may recommend one dose of potency 30 once a week before the due date, but only after 36–37 weeks gestation.

Other remedies that may be useful are:

- pulsatilla—useful when mother feels helpless, weepy or unable to cope
- chamomilla—for those women very sensitive to pain, especially if she has a furious temper and cannot be pleased!
- natrum mur—useful for backache in labour; may be used instead of Caulophyllum when labour is not proceeding because the mother feels inhibited, and is perhaps cross, sensitive and resentful about interference
- cimicifuga—this remedy may be needed when labour is not proceeding in cases where the mother is very nervous, and her pain and symptoms move around and change quickly, especially if there are also twitching, spasmodic movements
- gelsemium—for backache with drowsiness and weakness
- kali carb—for backache with irritability usually.

Midwives should refer to *The Midwife's Code of Practice*, paragraph 34 (UKCC 1994): 'The administration of homeopathic and herbal substances', which states: 'Homeopathic and herbal medicines are subject to the licensing provisions of the Medicines Act 1968 ...' and which provides a caution relating to products which were licensed without evaluation of their efficacy.

ACUPUNCTURE

Acupuncture is an ancient healing art which is regarded as conventional medicine in China and the Far East. Acupuncturists believe that health is dependent upon the correct flow of energy through meridians, which are invisible tracks running through the body (Fig. 8.2). Acupuncturists believe that the strength and clarity of these meridians govern the health of all of the vital organs in the body. Acupuncture aims to harmonise the body's energy system by stimulating the appropriate meridians using needles, heat, electricity or pressure.

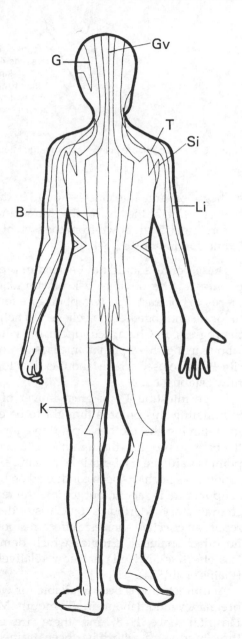
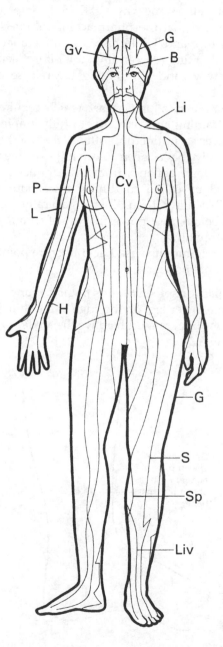

Figure 8.2   14 important meridians used in acupuncture.

Recent Western medical research has shown acupuncture to be effective in stimulating the release of endorphins, the body's natural pain-killers, and it seems to be capable of working as a powerful analgesic during labour. Acupuncture can help a woman in labour by reducing anxiety and fear, thereby reducing pain. It is believed to work in much the same way as TENS. Thompson (1988) reported that the pharmacological effects of acupuncture and TENS have certain similarities, i.e. inhibiting descending inhibitory neuronal pathways and stimulating the release of enkephalins.

Acupuncture is a precise art which requires extensive training and practice. To fully employ the resources acupuncture offers, the mother would ideally have been receiving treatment throughout her pregnancy from an acupuncturist who would be called in during the labour if required. 'Needling' the points is generally considered to be the most powerful way of stimulating the energy flow.

The most commonly used acupuncture points for labour are known as:

- 'sanyinjiao' or spleen 6—this point is found inside the lower leg, on the edge of the shin bone, four fingers' width above the ankle bone (Fig 8.3).

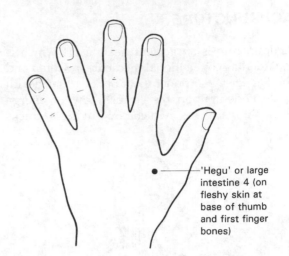

Figure 8.4   Acupuncture point: 'hegu' or large intestine 4.

- 'hegu' or large intestine 4—found in the fleshy skin at the base of the thumb and forefinger, 1 cm down from the web of thumb and forefinger (Fig. 8.4).

These points should not be used in pregnancy, because of the obvious risk of stimulating the uterus to contract. The two points are fairly easy to locate and together are believed to help labour to progress. In China, acupuncturists will induce labour using these points, in cases of postmaturity. It is also used where labour is slow to become fully established.

Large intestine 4 is a great mover of energy. Stimulating this point is thought to be excellent for relieving the mother's pain and for helping the baby to progress through the birth canal. This point is valuable if labour is advancing slowly.

Some research has been conducted on the use of acupuncture in labour, but to date the results are contradictory. Martoudis & Christofides (1990) report an effective analgesic effect in labour using no other analgesia. Studies which demonstrate less effective analgesia are now relatively dated (Wallis et al 1974).

Acupuncture has been available for women in pregnancy and labour in Plymouth Maternity Hospital since 1988, and there are currently three midwives who have been trained in the procedure. Budd (1995) describes the use of

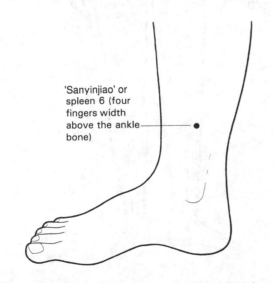
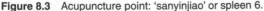

Figure 8.3   Acupuncture point: 'sanyinjiao' or spleen 6.

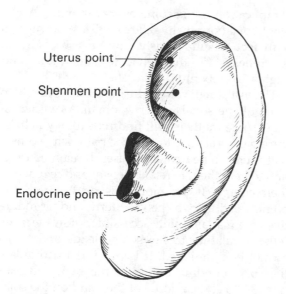

Uterus point

Shenmen point

Endocrine point

Figure 8.5 Acupuncture points on the ear as used in labour.

acupuncture points in the ear for labour (Fig. 8.5). Usually electro-acupuncture is used; needles are inserted in the ear at points which relate to the uterus, and have an effect on analgesia and relaxation of the body. Electrodes are attached to the needles, the controls are given to the mother so that she can 'turn the volume up or down' according to her pain levels at the time. The electro-acupuncture machine vibrates the needle, stimulating it more than if it were just resting in the ear. This technique has been developed through several years of experience by the midwife-acupuncturists at Plymouth and is currently being evaluated by them.

In China acupuncturists claim an 80% success rate at turning breech babies simply by applying moxibustion (a specific form of heat) to a point on the edge of the little toe, known as bladder 69; the optimum time for treatment is at around week 34 of pregnancy.

Acupuncture is particularly good at increasing a woman's stamina and general strength fairly quickly, and it may be helpful for a woman who is feeling very tired and depleted to consult an acupuncturist for treatment at about 36 weeks of pregnancy, once any possible medical condition has been excluded. Some mothers who have been

receiving acupuncture treatment during pregnancy have asked their acupuncturist to locate and mark the relevant points for their partner to stimulate (either by acupressure or by an electronic self-acupuncture device) during labour.

Acupressure is an alternative to needling which involves the use of pressure and massage at acupuncture points; it is therefore potentially a method more readily available for use in labour. However, there are as yet no reports of this method of treatment.

REFLEXOLOGY

Reflexology has been practised for thousands of years in China and Egypt, and was introduced to the West at the beginning of this century by Dr William Fitzgerald, who noted that pressure on specific areas of the body could have an anaesthetising effect on a related area. Developing his theory, he divided the body into 10 equal zones (Fig. 8.6). Doreen Bayly is well recognised as one of the main proponents of reflexology in the UK.

Further developments in reflexology techniques during the 1930s suggested that congestion in any part of the foot mirrored congestion or tension in a related part of the body. Today, reflexologists apply gentle pressure to the feet and hands to stimulate energy flow and to help restore the body's natural equilibrium. An experienced reflexologist will detect tiny crystalline deposits and tensions in the feet which block vital energy pathways, possibly resulting in illness.

Reflexology offers women in labour a very unobtrusive, gentle method of pain control. There are reflexes for the uterus, fallopian tubes, ovaries and pelvic region situated in the areas around the ankle bones which can be stimulated by massage (Fig. 8.7), using either circular movements with the thumb and forefinger or the press and hold method, similar to acupressure. There are also reflexes located in the hands; the specific points relating to the pelvic region are located at the wrists and base of the thumb.

It is often best to massage the whole foot once labour has commenced, to help relax the mother and to assist in relaxing and relieving any tension that may be held in the internal organs. Particular

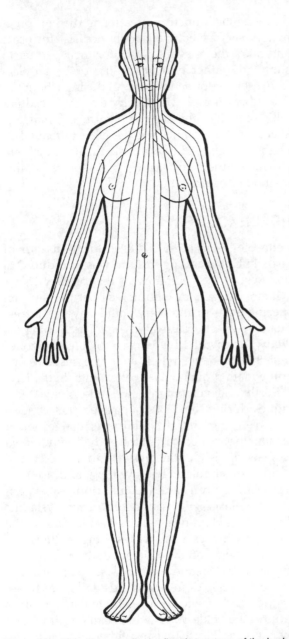

Figure 8.6 The 10 longitudinal reflexology zones of the body.

complications by keeping energy moving. At the height of labour many reflexologists will work on both feet simultaneously, applying pressure to the reflexes for the pelvic region, uterus and vagina for maximum pain relief.

The use of reflexology during labour is likely to be highly personal to every woman. As with massage, some mothers will find reflexology helpful during contractions to ease the pain, while others will prefer to be treated after each main contraction to help them to relax, recover and regenerate their energy. If the mother is on her feet, the points relating to the pelvis, uterus and reproductive organs are still accessible, however the reflexes relating to the solar plexus and lungs cannot be stimulated. It is possible to stimulate the corresponding points in the hands instead (Fig. 8.8), i.e. the middle of the hand on the solar plexus point for stress release, and just below the third finger for the lungs. Stimulating points on the ankles and wrists relating to the uterus is said to be very effective in initiating labour where an induction would otherwise be necessary.

HYPNOTHERAPY AND SELF-HYPNOSIS

Hypnosis, whether directed by the woman herself or by a therapist, is a combination of subtle and profound relaxation with potent and positive suggestion designed to command the mind to produce a specific result. Some studies have demonstrated the power of the mind on the body and have found hypnosis to be an effective method of inducing relaxation and controlling pain. One study examined the influence of hypnotherapy in pregnancy on the length of labour and the use of analgesia (Jenkins & Pritchard 1993). Although there were some methodological problems, the study suggests that hypnosis reduces the need for further analgesia. Hypnosis has been described as an 'altered state of consciousness in which a subject can gain a degree of control over bodily functions (e.g. perception of pain) not normally under conscious control' (Brann 1995).

In order for the woman to learn positive suggestion, she needs to be relaxed. This can be

focus may be given to the points relating to the solar plexus and the lungs, to help release stress and deepen the mother's breathing. As labour progresses, the points around the ankle bones relating to the pelvis, uterus and sacrum become a priority. These points will help to quicken the process of labour, relieve pain and help to reduce

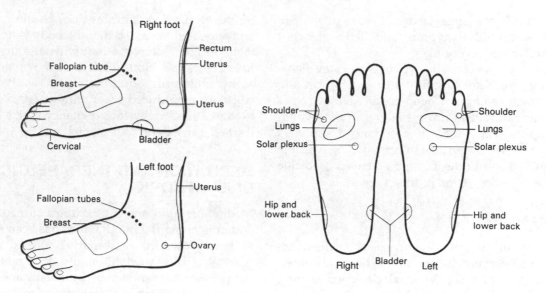

Figure 8.7   Reflexology points used in labour.

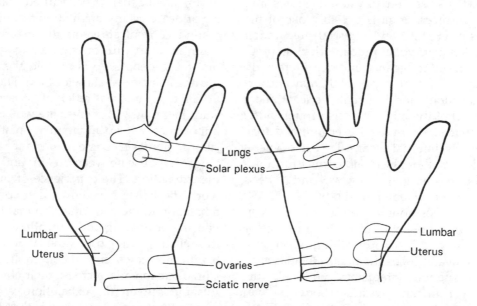

Figure 8.8   Reflexology points, including those which may be used in labour.

achieved very simply using a progressive muscle relaxation exercise, similar to the type of relaxation many midwives and physiotherapists teach in preparation for labour. Maximum confidence, relaxation and pain control may then be obtained throughout labour. If the mother wanted to use hypnosis specifically to control pain, she would be advised to consult an experienced hypnotherapist, who would teach her a self-hypnosis technique. Once the hypnotist has taught the woman how to move into a hypnotic state, she can put her self-hypnosis 'suggestion' on a tape and listen to her own voice giving the commands. Hypnosis is likely to be most effective when started early in labour. It is also suggested that some people are more susceptible to hypnosis; it will therefore not be effective for everyone.

There are several self-hypnosis tapes available to buy which are specifically directed at dealing with pain, and have been reported to be very helpful to mothers during labour. Most hypnotherapists will be able to recommend suppliers of quality tapes. Further information is available through the Institute of Complementary Medicine (refer to section at end of this chapter).

YOGA

Yoga is an ancient art and science which has evolved over centuries in India. There are numerous different types of yoga, all designed to bring balance to the body, mind and spirit. The most commonly practised yoga in the West is Hatha yoga, which focuses on physical postures and breathing practices. Yoga is possibly one of the best forms of exercise and physical preparation for birth. Regular yoga practice during pregnancy is believed to balance and distribute body fluids; calm the nervous system, thereby encouraging relaxation and mental concentration; strengthen all of the major muscle groups in the body without strain or over-exertion; and tone and balance the internal organs. There are several poses which are thought to aid correct functioning of the reproductive organs, and indeed almost any other system in the body.

Most of the positions or poses involve deep stretches, which are held quietly for a minute or so whilst focusing on the breathing which also serves to calm and focus the mind. Regular yoga practice throughout pregnancy will help the mother to get 'in tune' with her body, and can help to prevent headaches, morning sickness, fatigue and back pain, and ensure that she is in peak physical condition for labour.

It is very difficult to practice yoga whilst in labour, however many women, when opting for an active birth, find leaning forward onto a support, whilst sitting on their haunches with knees wide apart on the floor very helpful at relieving pain in the lower spine and pelvis. Yoga teachers believe that this position helps to take the weight off the uterus and spine, as does kneeling down on hands and knees, so that the body is horizontal to the floor. Many mothers will naturally gravitate to these positions if left to their own devices. Many childbirth educators, such as Balaskas (1989) have produced programmes of yoga-based exercises specifically for pregnancy which, when learned, can extend to use in labour.

MEDITATION AND THERAPEUTIC BREATHWORK

Meditation is an ancient technique for focusing and quietening the mind, which has been shown to have powerful rejuvenating effects on the body. Practising meditation and deep relaxation can release stress and tension, mentally and physically, and encourage the secretion of endorphins. Nothing could be more important for a mother during labour than to be 'centred', calm and feeling at peace. Many meditation techniques centre around concentrating on the breathing. Often, when in a stressful or frightening situation, the first thing people do is to hold their breath, or breathe in a very shallow fashion. The feeling is a little like an internal reflex of 'stop the world, I want to get off'. Midwives are well aware of the importance of deep and regular breathing during labour, however some expectant mothers are taught to pause between breaths and to push out the exhalation. The experience of many breathwork specialists has shown that connecting the inhalation to the exhalation, so that there is little pausing or holding of the breath, is a more natural, relaxing way to breathe. Working with the breath this way seems to help mothers to release stored tension and increase their ability to focus. Pushing out on the exhalation can sometimes lead to hyperventilation and is therefore not recommended. Gravity will take care of the exhalation, and most breathwork teachers encourage mothers to focus on deep inhalation only.

Other forms of meditation teach concentration on a word, mantra or positive statement which is repeated inwardly over and over again. This form of meditation is designed to concentrate and calm the mind, thereby dissipating fears and tension. Transcendental meditation (TM) works on this principle. Different methods will work for different people. There are countless meditation techniques to choose from. The midwife can help each mother to find an approach that works for her, and encourage her to practise using it well before the birth. The mother will then feel confident to use it from the onset of labour to help her centre on the task ahead and maintain her centre as she progresses to the more advanced stages of labour. Meditation and breathwork sessions taught either by the midwife or by an experienced meditation teacher can successfully enable the mother to identify and release her fears of giving birth, as any emotions around the event, conscious or unconscious, are likely to surface during labour. Any increase in the mother's emotions will create tension in her body, which could increase her pain.

Some women may find it extremely difficult to meditate or relax. It may be important for some to address certain fears they may have, for example, those that may occur as a result of previous traumatic birth experiences. Some midwives have now established counselling facilities for women who have had bad experiences and unresolved birth issues (Charles & Curtis 1994, Westley 1995). This aspect of midwifery care has been found to be very effective in helping women deal with a traumatic birth, and can therefore be valuable in overcoming the fears in any subsequent labour. Midwives can help women by discussing their previous experiences with them, by explaining exactly what happened, often by going through case notes with them, and by filling in the gaps in memory. Realising that they are not to blame for things happening as they did, these women can then overcome fears, negative thoughts and often nightmares.

HERBALISM

Herbalism is one of the oldest forms of medicine and is the parent of modern drug therapy. Herbalists believe that herbal remedies are time tested and that natural combinations of substances, as found in plants, work synergistically, in accordance with nature, to bring about balance in a person. The active ingredients of many medical drugs are extracted from plants and synthesised into drugs which exert a specific, powerful effect on the body. However, there are few drugs that do not have side-effects, whereas most herbs, taken under the guidance of a qualified medical herbalist, are relatively free from side-effects as it is said that nature has devised a balanced medicine for most ailments.

Herbalists believe that every person is biochemically unique, and will devise herbal remedies individual to every person's past history and constitution. Herbalism is an excellent way of strengthening and toning the body, and is believed to be helpful in strengthening the uterus, vagina and reproductive organs, and in increasing the mother's stamina, thus helping her to have an easier and less painful delivery. Stapleton (1995) points out that traditional medicine has been the main health source for 75% of the world's population in recent years. The World Health Organization in fact recommends the use of such health measures rather than developing a dependence on expensive and inappropriate modern drugs.

A remedy which can be given in the last month of pregnancy to strengthen, tone and relax the uterus is a combination of red raspberry, dong quai, black haw, squaw vine, cramp bark and blue cohosh. This combination of herbs would help to elasticise the vagina, cervix and pelvis and to strengthen the heart. It is believed that perineal tearing can be greatly reduced and even prevented by massaging the perineum daily with wheatgerm or almond oil, or even the contents of a vitamin E capsule 1 month before the birth. This may help to make the tissue around the vagina stronger and more elastic, facilitating the birth process. During labour, herbal remedies are reported to be of great benefit in relieving pain and helping to keep the mother calm and relaxed. Many herbalists recommend that, during labour, the mother sip a tea made up of skullcap, motherwort, chamomile, lindenblossom, pennyroyal and golden seal. The best way to take these herbs is to use one teaspoon of each herb made up into a tea, which is left to infuse for 15 minutes, adding some honey and lemon juice to improve the taste. In the immediate postnatal period many herbalists will recommend a combination of red raspberry and St John's wort to be taken as a tea for 6 weeks, to tone and balance the uterus and reproductive organs.

Once again, attention is drawn to *The Midwife's Code of Practice* (UKCC 1994, paragraph 34).

NATUROPATHY

Naturopathy can be best summed up by the quote from Hippocrates, father of modern medicine, who said: 'Let your food be your medicine, and your medicine be your food.' Modern naturopaths employ scientific research, as with other areas of complementary therapy, to corroborate the healing properties of natural foods, vitamins, minerals, dietary supplements and water therapy, to provide the optimum conditions for the body to function.

Naturopathy focuses heavily on the prevention of disease, rather than on cure. Naturopaths further believe that the standard recommended daily allowances (RDAs) of nutrients are not enough to maintain good health and prevent disease. Cheraskin & Ringford (1977) undertook a study of the dietary health and lifestyle of 13 500 people. They proposed that the healthiest individuals took supplements and ate a diet rich in nutrients relative to calories. The findings led to a concept of 'suggested optimal nutrient allowances' (SONAs) which give clear guidelines for the optimum intake of essential vitamins and minerals that are much higher than RDAs.

Food is nevertheless usually grown using modern farming methods on nutrient-depleted soil, sprayed with pesticides up to 20 times during the growing season, often picked too early, artificially ripened, and stored too long for it to retain even a fifth of its original nutrients. Eating organic food grown on nutrient rich soil may be a wise choice! However, for some women, the cost of such good nutritive food may prove prohibitive.

Midwives and health professionals will be aware of the need for optimum nutrition before conception for both mother and father, and during pregnancy for the mother, in order to safeguard the future health of the baby. Naturopaths will specifically advise the woman in pregnancy to exclude from her diet what are known as 'anti-nutrients'—including tea, coffee, refined carbohydrates, sugar, alcohol and cigarettes—and to eat fresh vegetables (especially greens), fruit, whole grains, lentils and pulses, nuts and seeds, live yoghurt, fish, free range eggs, farm cheese and meat—in that order. There are some vitamins and minerals that a naturopath may suggest as being helpful for maintaining energy levels and nutrition in labour, such as vitamin B complex, calcium, magnesium and vitamin E. A woman who approaches labour in an optimum state of health is more likely to progress normally, thus minimising pain.

SUMMARY

It is apparent that the basis of many complementary therapies is to reduce stress and anxiety, to increase relaxation and also increase the individual's personal involvement in their care. This does not mean that these therapies are any less effective than traditional medicine for that reason. If the woman's physical, psychological, social and spiritual needs are addressed throughout treatment, this would present a truly holistic form of care. Many of the therapies based in oriental medicine address spirituality explicitly, arguably adding to the psychological effect.

Mason (1995) emphasises some key factors for the provision of aromatherapy, which is perhaps applicable to all forms of care and complementary therapies which every midwife should consider: 'We live in a multicultural society and it should be feasible that we can offer honest and informed choices to women … the ideal holistic service should be non-prejudiced and non-racist, affordable and freely available, no matter what the socio-economic status is of the women who seek it.' The point here is that some women may not have access to some forms of complementary therapy because of limited finances, or they may be living in an area where there is no practising therapist. It is therefore suggested that midwives and complementary therapists should work together to increase access to therapy in pregnancy and labour, and to increase availability through the health services which must ultimately benefit all women in childbirth.

Finally, midwives should draw attention to their overall responsibility in relation to their practice through the UKCC's (1992) code of professional conduct:

'As a registered nurse, midwife or health visitor, you are personally accountable for your practice and, in the exercise of your professional accountability, must:

1. act always in such a manner as to promote and safeguard the interests and well being of patients and clients

2. ensure that no action or omission on your part, or within your sphere of responsibility, is detrimental to the interests, condition or safety of patients and clients

3. maintain and improve your professional knowledge and competence

4. acknowledge any limitations in your knowledge and competence and decline any duties or responsibilites unless able to perform them in a safe and skilled manner, and

5. work in an open and cooperative manner with patients, clients and their families, foster their independence and recognise and respect their involvement in the planning and delivery of care.'

REFERENCES

Balaskas J 1989 New active birth: a concise guide to natural childbirth. Thorsons, London

Brann L 1995 The role of hypnosis in obstetrics Diplomate. The Journal of Diplomates of the Royal College of Obstetricians and Gynaecologists 2 (2): 95–99

Budd S 1992 Traditional Chinese medicine in obstetrics. Midwives Chronicle and Nursing Notes 105 (1): 140–143

Budd S 1995 Acupuncture. In: Tiran D, Mack S (eds) Complementary therapies for pregnancy and childbirth. Bailliere Tindall, London

Cheraskin E, Ringsdorff WM 1977 Predictive medicine: a study in strategy - a plan for maintaining health by avoiding disease. Keats

Charles J, Curtis C 1994 Birth afterthoughts: a listening service. British Journal of Midwifery 2 (7): 331–334

Department of Health 1993 Changing childbirth. HMSO, London

Jenkins M W, Pritchard M H 1993 Hypnosis: practical applications and theoretical considerations in normal labour. British Journal of Obstetrics and Gynaecology 100 (3): 221–226.

Martoudis S, Christofides K 1990 Electroacupuncture for pain relief in labour. Acupuncture and Electrotherapeutics Research 2: 105

Mason M 1995 A fertile partnership; the role of aromatherapy in midwifery. Aromatherapy Quarterly 47: 27–29

Stapleton H 1995 Women as midwives and herbalists. In: Tiran D, Mack S (eds) Complementary therapies for pregnancy and childbirth. Bailliere Tindall, London

Stevenson C 1992 Orange blossom evaluation. International Journal of Aromatherapy 4(3): 22–24

Tiran D 1995 Massage and aromatherapy. In: Tiran D, Mack S (eds) Complementary therapies for pregnancy and childbirth. Bailliere Tindall, London

Thompson J W 1988 Pharmacology of transcutaneous electrical nerve stimulation. Intractable Pain Society 7 (1): 33–40

UKCC 1992 Standards for the administration of medicines. UKCC, London

UKCC 1993 Midwives' rules. UKCC, London

UKCC 1994 The midwife's code of practice. UKCC, London

Wallis L, Schnider S, Palahnuik R, Spivey H 1974 An evaluation of acupuncture analgesia in obstetrics. Anaesthesiology 41 (6): 596

Webb P 1992 Homeopathy for midwives and pregnant women. British Homeopathic Association, London

Westley W 1995 Quoted in: Woman on Sunday, Sunday Mercury, May 28, p 23

FURTHER INFORMATION

The Institute of Complementary Medicine
PO Box 194
London
SE16 1QZ
Tel: 0171 237 5165.

The Aromatherapy Organisations Council
3 Latymer Close
Braybrooke
Market Harborough
Leicester
LE16 8LN
Tel/Fax: 01858 434242

British Homeopathic Association
27a Devonshire Street
London
W1N 1RJ
Tel: 0171 9352163

The School of Herbal Medicine
Bucksteep Manor
Bodle Street Green
Nr Hailsham
East Sussex
Tel: 01323 833812/4

'Herbline' (information available from a qualified herbal practitioner Tuesdays, Wednesdays and Fridays):
01323 832858

The National Institute of Medical Herbalists
Tel: 01392 426 022
or the General Council and register of Consultant Herbalists
01243 267126.

For information about training in homeopathy:
Society of Homeopaths
2 Artisan Road
Northampton
NN1 4HU
Tel: 01604 21400.

To order homeopathic medicines and literature contact
Ainsworths Homeopathic Pharmacy : 0171 935 5330

British Acupuncture Council
Park House
206–208 Latimer Road
London
W10 6RE
Tel: 0181 9640222; fax: 0181 9640333.

The Association of Reflexologists
27 Old Gloucester St
London
WC1 3XX.

Pat Morrell: who practises a unique form of reflexology;
works with women in pregnancy and childbirth, and
provides training in Morrell reflexology:
Reflexology School and Clinic
Sedbury Park Lodge
Sedbury
Nr Chepstow
Gwent
NP6 7EY

Institute of Optimum Nutrition
Tel: 0181 877 9993

9

Water in labour

Fiona Alderdice and Sally Marchant

LEARNING OUTCOMES

At the end of this chapter the reader will have

- **an increased awareness of current research findings relating to the use of water for pain relief in labour and the work of the National Perinatal Epidemiology Unit, Oxford**

- **an increased understanding of some of the implications of the use of water in labour**

- **a brief introduction to the historical context of the use of water in labour**

- **considered the pain relieving effect of water**

- **increased confidence in advising on the use of water in labour based on evidence to date**

- **an appreciation of the need for further research into the use of water in labour and its effect on pain modulation.**

Pain relief in labour has been of great interest to women, care-givers and participants in the birth process for centuries. It is an ongoing quest for agents which can offer relief from the pain of labour and birth without unacceptable risks or side-effects. Research into methods of pain relief offered to women should feature prominently in health services, to provide women with a realistic choice of options. Information available to women should come from tested evidence, so that those involved with caring and advising about methods of pain relief in labour can feel secure that the advice they give and the care they practise is sound, practical and safe.

This chapter looks at the use of water for pain relief in labour. It is intended to give the reader more information about the background to the use of water, and to help practitioners to feel better equipped to advise on the use of water for labour and/or for birth. It is not intended as a manual of instruction on the specific care for clinical practice, as we would argue that there is much more research needed in this area. The information given is mainly in the context of specially provided birthing pools but there is also reference to the use of conventional baths for labour (and occasionally for birth), and the use of showers. When labour takes place in a bath or pool this is a very different environment from most conventional labour settings on 'dry land'. As the water surrounds the mother the effects of this might be more widespread than other forms of pain relief, both those given systemically and those applied locally. Evaluation or assessment of the effects of the use of water for the relief of pain cannot be easily isolated from other procedures and practices used to care for women in all forms of birth settings, both conventional and alternative.

In looking at any beneficial or harmful effects of using water for pain relief in labour it is therefore difficult to separate the effects of the water from those other practices and procedures associated with the different management. Some of these may be common to conventional practice but others may be quite different. Further research should aim to tease out the implications of these differences so that studies looking at the effect of water will be reliable and the method will therefore be more likely to be adopted as one of the options available for women and will be offered by a wider group of care-givers.

We will look at the possible benefits and risks associated with immersion in water for pain relief in labour and for birth, and give information about midwives' current practice. The research evidence presently available will be explored and suggestions will be made about where further research in this area is needed. The majority of the information is based on a national survey of labour and birth in water which was undertaken by the National Perinatal Epidemiology Unit (NPEU) in Oxford to provide a picture of national practice in England and Wales (Alderdice 1995a). Later on in the chapter we give practical information about offering labour and/or birth in water to women as a choice, using the experiences of a hospital where birth in water is now part of routine midwifery care (E Burns 1995, pers. comm.).

THE HISTORY OF IMMERSION IN WATER

Bathing in warm water is widely perceived as beneficial, being said to aid relaxation and reduce stress. Although the use of water for pain relief in labour and as an environment for birth has only recently attracted attention as a possible choice for women, its use in pregnancy and labour is not a new practice, with the first report of a birth under water being published in 1805 (Cammu et al 1992).

In this century conventional baths in labour have been used where maternity care has been provided, whether this was in a hospital or community setting. In the NPEU survey one midwife reflects: 'I am old enough to remember baths on admission to hospital and women stayed in them longer than necessary for hygiene ... I suspect this has been happening "since Adam was a lad".'

The growth in popularity and also in the use of birthing pools revolves mostly around the work of childbirth pioneers such as Leboyer and Odent. Michel Odent (1983) described the first birth which took place underwater in Pithiviers in 1983, and both he and Leboyer emphasise the need for birth to be gentle and more natural in its progress (Leboyer 1991). This shift in emphasis is also viewed as part of the process of returning more control of the birth to the mother, to make the event less traumatic for all those involved. Where water is used for the labour environment, the mother is most likely to be immersed in a receptacle which is large enough to allow her some mobility within the water. Such receptacles are now commonly referred to as birthing pools although they vary considerably in design, shape and capacity.

Using water in a bath or pool is thought to facilitate the physiological progress of labour, possibly to make it shorter, and to reduce the use of analgesic drugs with ongoing benefits for the new-born baby. In his 1983 case series, Odent described the use of water for birth in 100 women. Many women in the hospital at Pithiviers used the pool for pain relief in labour, but some women were then unable to leave the pool for the delivery. The babies were subsequently delivered while the mother was still in the water—no adverse outcomes were observed for mother or baby.

The work of Odent has attracted considerable attention over the last decade and other prominent figures in the field of childbirth have promoted a renewed interest in the use of water for labour and more recently for the actual birth. The choice of a labour and/or birth in water was initially more likely to be available to those women who had opted for private care from independent practitioners. In recent years an increasing number of women using mainstream NHS maternity services have requested the use of water for labour and/or birth, and resources have been made available to provide this, alongside other methods of pain relief and management for labour. The use of water, particularly in labour, is now viewed in a different light from the more usual advice given to women in early labour, where they are told to get into a (conventional) bath in the belief that it will bring comfort and increase relaxation.

A climate of growing dissatisfaction with the standardised care offered to women by the maternity services resulted in the Department of Health (England) publishing the policy document *Changing Childbirth* (Department of Health 1993). This supports the philosophy of returning to women more freedom of choice (and information on which to make that choice), and identifies the use of water during labour as an example of this. The report recommends better provision and access to birthing pools for women within the NHS in England.

With this background, women may find the idea of using a birthing pool attractive, not just for labour but for the birth itself, because of the possible advantages of reduced pain and a more 'intervention-free' form of childbirth. Those

involved in intrapartum care—midwives, consultant obstetricians and GPs—are being faced with increasing numbers of requests from women for a practice that they may feel ill-prepared for, as well as having doubts over its safety and effectiveness.

EFFECTS OF WATER
Pain relief

The theory that water relieves the pains of labour remains untested, although there are several hypothetical suggestions of the way in which warm water might act. One theory stems from an empirical belief (Lederman et al 1978) that warm water surrounding the body, as in a bath, soothes cutaneous nerve endings, causing vasodilatation in the skin and relaxation of tiny muscles in the hair follicles, and generally reduces stress in labour. Simpkin (1989) suggests that water has beneficial effects which can be accounted for by the gate-control theory of pain relief:

By reducing stress in labour, the bath enhances the woman's sense of well-being and reduces her pain perception. The higher brain centres (thalamus and cortex) send inhibitory impulses to the dorsal column to inhibit transmission of pain signals. Thermal receptors and tactile receptors are activated by immersion in water and more so by the spray of a shower or the swirling water of the whirlpool bath. Thus, the dorsal column receives stimuli from all over the periphery, and the gate to pain is closed, inhibiting transmission of those impulses to the cortex.

Other possible effects

Other possible effects in addition to non-pharmacological pain relief have been cited in the literature.

Altered pace of labour. It is suggested that acceleration of labour may occur in relation to the degree of cervical dilatation on entry to the pool. Odent (1983) suggests, from observations in his case series, that cervical dilatation of 5 cm should be attained and that this is then the best time for the labouring woman to get into the pool to accelerate labour. However, it is also thought that immersion can space out the contractions with the effect of slowing down the labour. Alternatively, Zimmerman et al (1993) advise that immersion in warm water is best in the early stages if it is to have the most positive effect on dilation. There is therefore a lack of agreement in the stated effects of the use of water in labour, and further information appears to be needed in order for these effects to be not only unequivocal, but also of use to clinicians who wish to advise women on the best use of water in labour.

Lowering of blood pressure. Taking a bath in pregnancy has been shown to lower blood pressure (Doniec-Ulman et al 1987) and it is suggested that a similar effect may occur in labour. Rosenthal (1991) reports that women who develop arterial hypertension during labour (but who are free from other manifestations of toxaemia) have a dramatic, significant reduction in blood pressure within 2 minutes of entering the pool.

Reduced perineal trauma. Although reduced perineal trauma has been reported for women giving birth in water (Burns & Greenish 1993, Garland & Jones 1994), it is unclear whether any reduction in perineal trauma is related to the effects of water on the perineum or to lack of intervention during the delivery. For example, it may be more difficult for midwives to perform an episiotomy underwater; and furthermore there are issues of possible bias because women who use the pool for birth are selected in some way as eligible and, as such, may have specific characteristics which are different from the total population. Further research is needed to assess this.

Emotional advantage. The use of specially designed birthing pools for labour, rather than conventional baths, offers the woman an environment in which she can be much more mobile, as the water lessens the effect of gravity on the body and the space gives her room to move about. She is also likely to have greater control over her environment, with the possible decrease in interventions leading to a better emotional experience without compromising a healthy fetal outcome.

Possible risks

Infection. There is thought to be an increased risk of infection, and cases of infection and the potential for infection for both mothers and babies have been identified and reported following the use of a birthing pool (Rawal et al 1994, Hawkins 1995). Uncovered skin lesions, faeces in the water or the presence of other people in the water all contribute to the risk of infection for the mother and baby as well as for professional and lay birth attendants.

Inhalation of water by new-born. During the birth, fluid is squeezed out of the fetal lungs by compression in the birth canal. The lungs are therefore optimally prepared for breathing air. In uncomplicated labour babies have an inhibitory reflex which reduces the likelihood of them taking a breath until exposed to an appropriate stimulus, such as air, a colder temperature or touch. There is concern that babies who are metabolically compromised from the conditions of the labour and delivery will try to breathe as soon as the head is delivered, thus overriding the inhibitory reflex—if this occurs underwater then water may be inhaled (Walker 1994).

Water embolism. Odent (1983) described a theoretical risk to the mother of water embolism if the placenta was delivered underwater. He does not give any physiological background to this but the concept may be based on the possible but rare occurrence of a foreign substance entering the woman's circulation during separation of the placenta from the uterine wall. Where births take place on dry land this foreign substance is usually amniotic fluid, but can be air, and it is said to be associated with forceful contractions producing a form of negative pressure. The embolus will travel to the lungs where it will block the smaller blood vessels, preventing the transference of oxygen to the blood from the lung spaces. This will result in respiratory distress, the severity of the respiratory problem depending on the size of the embolus. At its most severe it can result in sudden death, however more common manifestations are tachypnoea, tachycardia and cyanosis. To date the possibility of water entering the maternal circulation in this way remains a theoretical risk and we are not aware of any reported cases.

Increased blood loss. Estimating the amount of blood loss is also problematic, during labour as well as after the birth, and when estimating blood loss under water it is difficult to be accurate, although this has not received very much attention (Balaskas & Gordon 1992, Harmsworth 1994). As warmth induces hyperaemia and has a relaxing effect on the uterine muscles, it is suggested that this could possibly lead to an increase in blood loss after delivery of the placenta (Zimmerman et al 1993).

Delay in emergencies. There are also concerns about the ability to assist the mother if there is a need for her to get out of the pool quickly. This could arise from the need to expedite the delivery by, perhaps, an operative procedure, where shoulder dystocia has occurred, or in cases of obvious haemorrhage or collapse of the mother. It is suggested that there is both a greater risk of accident and injury to the woman and the birth attendants in these circumstances and a substantial delay should an urgent intervention be required (Zimmerman et al 1993).

THE EVIDENCE

Most of the information available about labour and birth in water is anecdotal and many of the published case reports and case series will be referred to throughout the chapter.

Randomised trials

The most reliable data on any practice is obtained through the mounting and reporting of results of randomised controlled trials. Currently, results of three small randomised controlled trials of labour in water are available (Bastide 1992, Schorn et al 1993, Cammu et al 1994). These studies allow for the assessment of the effect of immersion in water on various outcomes, such as length of labour and pain perception, while minimising the biasing effects of the mother's age, parity and other variables. Caution should still be exercised in the inferences made from these studies which are necessarily based on low-power calculations.

Bastide (1992). In this study, 295 women were recruited, 152 to the 'bath group' and 143 to 'conventional care'. The outcome measures were the number of times and duration of bath use,

comparison of the duration of the different stages of labour, and the presence of any complications. Bastide found that 70% of women used the pool only once, the mean time in the bath being 27 minutes. The mean duration of labour, particularly in the first stage, was longer when using a bath. Despite the lengthened labour, both women and staff were unanimous in claiming the benefits of the bath for comfort and relaxation. No complications were associated specifically with bath use.

Schorn et al (1993). These authors studied 93 women between 36 and 41 weeks' gestation, with no major obstetric or medical complications in active labour and with membranes intact. A total of 45 women were in the 'water immersion' group and 48 were in the 'no water immersion' group. Women in the 'water immersion' group used a hot tub with air jets and were encouraged to stay in for as long as they wanted; they also had control of the water temperature. Once out of the pool they could use other methods of pain relief. Women in the 'no water immersion' group used a full range of other methods of pain relief, which included use of a shower but excluded water immersion. The study assesses a wide range of outcomes, which include the rate of cervical dilatation, the length of the first and second stages of labour, the method of delivery, the condition of the infant assessed by Apgar scores, the neonatal weight and any presence of infection. Their results conclude that water immersion did not affect the rate of cervical dilation, contraction pattern, length of labour or use of analgesia. They also found no evidence of increased maternal or neonatal morbidity, which included no increase in infection.

Cammu et al (1994). In this study, 110 nulliparous low risk women in spontaneous labour were recruited. A total of 54 women used a bath, and 56 were in the control group. The effects of up to 50–60 minutes immersion in water were assessed. Labour pain perception was measured using a visual analogue scale for both the groups. No significant difference was found for labour pain perception based on these scores, and there was also no difference in the use of epidural analgesia, labour duration, frequency of operative deliveries or neonatal complications. From the participants' view, however, those who had used the bath reported greater satisfaction than those in the control group.

Trials in progress. Three randomised controlled trials of labour in water are still in progress (Rydhstrom 1992, Rush 1992, Nickodem 1995, pers. comm.). The trial being conducted by Rydhstrom in Sweden will have a sample of over 1000 participants and the main aim is to test whether immersion during labour increases the risk of admission to a neonatal unit. In Rush's study a total sample of 800 is being sought and the main aim is to assess the effect of immersion in water on pain and progress in labour. This much-needed data from larger studies will hopefully provide a clearer picture of the benefits and hazards of using water for labour and/or birth.

A randomised controlled trial of birth in water is currently underway in South Africa. This trial looks at perineal trauma and neonatal outcome as the main outcome measures, as well as looking at the views of the women from a physically subjective perspective. The total sample size aims to be 120 low risk multiparous women, and participants are asked to complete two questionnaires, the first within 24 hours of delivery and the second at 6 weeks postnatally.

Preliminary analysis of 54 subjects shows an overall trend (the numbers are too small for meaningful statistical analysis at this point) for those women allocated to give birth in water to have more favourable physical subjective outcomes. Examples of these trends are that the women who gave birth in water experienced less pain both in labour and 24 hours post-delivery, and expressed greater satisfaction with their ability to cope in the second stage. There were no differences in neonatal outcome, and birth canal trauma was similar in both groups (experimental group, 27%; control group, 26%). Episiotomy was performed slightly more often in the control group. More in-depth statistical analysis will be undertaken on completion of recruitment (C. Nickodem 1995, pers. comm.).

Non-randomised trials

Useful information can also be obtained from non-randomised cohort studies. The data from these studies are less reliable as there is more chance of bias in the sample. They also tend to be retrospective, so data are more likely to be incomplete or unreliable. In the following section we refer to five non-randomised cohort studies which have been published (Lenstrup et al 1987, Waldenstrom & Nilsson 1992, Burns & Greenish 1993, Garland & Jones 1994, Hawkins 1995).

Details of the size and main results of these studies can be found in Table 9.1. All the authors highlighted that the women studied had to fulfil a number of criteria which suggested they were likely to have an uncomplicated pregnancy and labour.

Conclusions from trials

Reviewing these results collectively, the effects of immersion in water during labour and/or birth are still unclear. To obtain clear and reliable data a large multi-centred randomised controlled trial is needed. The present studies are too small and, in the case of the cohort studies, too open to bias for reliable data to be provided. Further research is currently being considered to look at the feasibility of mounting a randomised control study in the UK.

In the absence of substantive research the clinical experience of others becomes paramount (Odent 1983, Sidenblah 1983, Church 1989). However, care based predominantly on practice and beliefs has many potential problems. Contradictory approaches begin to emerge, and without clear evidence it may be hard for professionals and consumers to choose between them. Also, it is impossible to say whether or not the practice is beneficial or safe based on the experience alone. Where complications arise which are rare, individual experience will not be sufficient to identify the possible causes or implications. Even where practice is subject to clinical audit it is unlikely that this is sufficiently systematic to identify what may be common problems. Where personal experience of an event or events is recounted, this is likely to be substantially influenced by pre-existing beliefs in the benefits or otherwise of the practice, and recall may be exaggerated or minimised according to the preferred option of the observer. All these effects apply to

Table 9.1   Details of non-randomised cohort studies

Authors	Intervention assessed	Number of women studied	Main results
Lenstrup et al (1987)	Immersion in water in 1st stage of labour for a maximum of 2 hours	• Pool group, $n =88$ • Control group, $n =72$	• Significantly fewer babies in pool group given supplementary formula • No other significant differences
Waldenstrom & Neilsson (1992)	Immersion in water for the 1st stage of labour	• Water group, $n =89$ • Control group, $n =89$	• Women in control group used significantly more analgesia • Babies born more than 24 hours after rupture of membranes had significantly lower 5-minute Apgars in the pool group. No other statistically significant differences detected
Burns & Greenish (1993)	Immersion in water during 1st and/or 2nd stage of labour	• Water group, $n =302$ • Control group, $n =302$	• More second degree tears in women using water but fewer episiotomies • Less supplementary analgesia use by women in water group
Garland & Jones (1994)	Immersion in water during 1st and/or 2nd stage of labour	• First stage water, $n =164$ • Waterbirth, $n =237$ • Control group, $n =257$	• Increase in incidence of second degree tears in waterbirth group but increase in incidence of intact genital tracts • More Apgars over 6 in waterbirth group • Shorter labours when a waterbirth group was compared to a non-immersion group
Hawkins (1995)	Immersion during the 2nd stage of labour	• Waterbirth group, $n =16$ • Control group, $n =16$	• Most women showed no sign of clinical infection • *Pseudomonas aeruginosa* and *Acinetobacter* sp. isolated from the water of one delivery

any innovation of technology or new practice and are particularly relevant for the use of water in a birthing pool or equivalent.

Where provider units offer the use of a birthing pool, as with other innovations, this choice is likely to be offered within a 'safety net' of certain risk factor conditions drawn up by professional care-givers. This framework might be said to help those responsible for care in labour to resolve the problems of safety, by giving the choice of using water in labour and/or for birth only to those women whom they anticipated, based on certain criteria, had a low risk of any complications.

Selection of women who may be eligible to use this option results in any experiential data being drawn from an unrepresentative sample of 'low risk' women and as such it cannot be reliably compared with the general population of labouring women. Therefore, to comment on the benefits and hazards of this practice a comparable group of 'low risk' women must be examined. This is more difficult than perhaps expected in

that the definition of 'low risk' and the components of pre-determined criteria remain open to interpretation and dispute.

A national survey of labour and birth in water

The lack of substantive research on immersion in water leads to the need for large prospective research studies to look into the effects of water for labour and for birth. As part of the ongoing programme of research into evaluating the effectiveness of care for pregnancy, childbirth and the neonatal period, the National Perinatal Epidemiology Unit was given funding from the Department of Health to survey the use of water in provider units in England and Wales, and to use this information to facilitate further research in this area. The national survey (England and Wales) had the following aims, all of which apply to the provision and practice of labouring and/or giving birth in water:

- to describe the extent and types of options available
- to estimate the number of women who laboured and/or gave birth in water in 1992 and 1993
- to collect information on policies for birthing pool use, of local evaluations and resource implications for the health service
- to assess the feasibility of further research
- to assess the extent of reported problems for mothers, babies and midwives.

Method

The survey was carried out between August 1993 and June 1994 and each provider unit in England and Wales ($n = 219$) was initially contacted using a postal questionnaire. A contact in each provider unit was nominated to take part in a structured telephone interview. This person was usually someone who had information about the local policies and practice associated with the use of water for labour and/or birth. The respondents were asked for information related to the use of water, both in a pool and in a conventional bath, to include any problems encountered for mothers, babies and midwives in both hospital and community settings.

A total of 195 (89%) units reported some type of birthing pool use past or present. The data on birthing pool practice were analysed only for the 102 provider units where more than four births in water had occurred over the 2-year period of study, 1992–1993. This was done in an attempt to reflect contemporary and actual clinical practice as described to us by respondents. We were interested to document what the midwives most commonly undertook as part of their clinical care, rather than to record their theoretically based knowledge of what was planned to take place in the form of written guidelines where they had little practical experience. We also wished to minimise the amount of anecdotal information.

A total of 217 (99%) units reported the use of water in a conventional bath. Questions related to conventional bath practice were not as detailed. As the practice was perceived as informal, details

regarding any record keeping or audit were rarely available—records of usage were not kept and practice was seen as largely unsupported by any particular policies, criteria or guidelines. The results of this study have been published in detail elsewhere (Alderdice et al 1995a, 1995b, Marchant et al, unpubl. data). For information in this chapter we are mainly using data from the NHS provider units when discussing details of practice. We hope that the information from the survey and subsequent discussion around these practice data will increase the existing exchange of information and ideas between those units already undertaking this practice on a large scale and those perhaps just embarking on it.

What is a birthing pool?

From the NPEU survey what was defined as a birthing pool appeared to depend on the perceived purpose of use. For example many hospitals had large baths; some preferred to see these as conventional baths, whereas others defined them as a birthing pool to be used for births as well as for labour. Many hospitals provided specially designed pools of different shapes and colours, and frequently set these into rooms decorated to reflect themes of water and relaxation. Where pools were not a permanent fixture, companies specialising in birthing pools and equipment offered special arrangements for both individual women and provider units.

It is usual for birthing pools to be large enough to allow the woman sufficient mobility when in the pool and to be of sufficient depth for the water to cover her abdomen, preferably up to the shoulders. This ensures maximum buoyancy and personal space for the mother. Also if a birth is planned in the pool, the greater depth means it is less likely for the mother to accidentally raise herself out of the water and expose the emerging baby to air before delivery of the body is complete. Such exposure is likely to trigger the response to take a gasp and the baby might take a breath whilst under, or partially under, the water. Complete immersion, by minimising the exposure to external stimuli reduces this possibility.

Caring for a woman using a birthing pool

In the NPEU study the most common ways midwives prepared themselves to assist women to use immersion in water were by the traditional resources of literature reviews, special interest group meetings and study days. In addition to these resources, several units set up an informal network to collaborate with neighbouring provider units or other units known to be undertaking the practice. Some of these units would act in an advisory capacity, while for other units this collaboration took the form of organising visits so that midwives could observe labours and births in water as well as exchanging information about guidelines, policies and procedures. For some units where the use of water especially for births was infrequent, midwives commented that gaining practical experience could be a problem and in some cases a few midwives acted as 'mentors' for others as they gained confidence.

Attendance by care-givers during labour and birth

All units ($n = 102$) said that a minimum of two midwives would be present for a birth in water. For attendance in labour it was normal for the majority of the units to have only one midwife, but 25% of units said that two midwives would normally be present throughout the labour. Constant supervision of women in both conventional baths and birthing pools is seen as essential (Scheller & Terinde 1994).

Who can use a birthing pool?

A number of hospitals that have accumulated considerable experience of using a birthing pool have, over the past few years, published details of their criteria and guidelines for use in various papers (Burns & Greenish 1993, Garland & Jones 1994, Nightingale 1994, Reid 1994). There was little variation within the NPEU survey on which women were considered suitable to use a birthing pool, mainly because of the circumstances of their pregnancy, as well as their past and current health. It was most common to describe the requirements in the criteria as fulfilling a 'low risk'. Certain criteria

regarding the condition of the mother when she was admitted in labour were identified as having to be met. These included an uncomplicated pregnancy, no medical complications, spontaneous onset of labour, and the need for a normal reading from a cardiotocograph when admitted in labour and prior to getting into the pool.

The elements of assessment for low risk remain subject to debate, and this was also reflected by some units which had only a few mandatory requirements as part of the formal criteria and otherwise expressed much greater flexibility depending on the mother, midwife and obstetrician involved. A further option for women and care-givers was the use of the birthing pool for labour only for those women identified as having a higher level of risk. There is a contradiction here, as there is little, if any evidence to support the classification of risk for women into high or low risk, and then relate this risk to the option to use water for labour only, or for both labour and the birth. Twins and breech deliveries have been reported in water (Lines 1993, Y Gordon 1994, pers. comm.), but these tend to be exceptions and not recommended practice.

Women should be informed that use of a birthing pool is a possibility, as well as the criteria for eligibility where present, and this information should be available to them in the antenatal period. A woman may be disappointed and distressed to find out at the last minute that she cannot use the pool for labour and/or birth. It is therefore important that women are fully informed of the circumstances when their chosen option may not be available.

The use of practice guidelines

We found in the NPEU survey that for a number of the hospitals who were offering labour and/or birth in water on a regular basis, the guidelines which they had drawn up had become 'gold standards' for a number of units across England and Wales. This appears to have led to some practices being regarded as the 'correct' procedures to adopt with little evaluation of their effectiveness.

An example of this is the guidance on the temperature of the water both for labour and for the birth. Where the 'gold standard' of a centre commonly using immersion in water has been adopted by another unit, there is often replication of the guidance on temperature control and/or the range of minimum and maximum water temperatures. This may be the case in spite of there being a number of other possible variations, for example the make of the pool, whether it is fixed or hired, the depth of water used, or what is used to measure the water temperature.

There must be a question mark over the safety of a provider unit adopting another unit's standard guidelines—which are based on empirical evidence from that unit—in the absence of any other evaluation or testing. Although this sharing of common practices may be beneficial, it is important for each provider unit to evaluate their own practice guidelines and for these in time to be based on research evidence for effectiveness and safety.

Considerations when assisting a woman labouring in a birthing pool

When using a birthing pool for pain relief in labour it is apparent that a number of key issues need to be taken into consideration. In the light of current knowledge the temperature of the water, the potential risks of infection, appropriate monitoring of the condition of the mother and fetus and the use of additional pain relief are central to the safe use of a birthing pool for labour and/or for birth.

Measuring water temperature. There are concerns about the effects on the fetus in pregnancy (Waldenstrom 1994) and during labour in water (Rosevear et al 1993) of exposing the mother to increased body temperature. Rosevear et al reported two adverse outcomes following labour in water and they suggested that thermoregulation changes occur in the baby with each degree of temperature rise after 34°C. They suggested that this could lead to increased fetal cerebral vasodilation, raised metabolic rate and subsequent increased oxygen requirements. A number of temperature recommendations have been provided (Rosevear et al 1993, Royal College of Midwives 1994, National Childbirth Trust 1995).

In practice, all but three of the provider units examined in the NPEU study measured the water temperature of the birthing pool, usually with a bath thermometer or thermostatic probe. Ninety-five percent had temperature recommendations of between 33 and 40°C, with the majority recommending between 36 and 38°C. In those units where a recommended temperature range was not stated, the temperature was kept either at body temperature or at a temperature that was 'comfortable for the mother' (Marchant et al, unpubl. data).

The risk of infection. Cases of infection following the use of a birthing pool have been reported (Rawal et al 1994, Alderdice et al 1995a, Hawkins 1995). There is no evidence available to support an increased risk, although two randomised controlled trials (Schorn et al 1993, Cammu et al 1994) have suggested that there is no difference between women labouring in water and controls; these results must be viewed with caution as the conclusions are drawn from small samples which might affect the statistical inferences made. The most frequent means of testing reported to us in the survey was for swabs to be taken from the equipment such as the outlet pipes and water pumps, for water samples to be taken, and, in some units, for routine swabs to be taken from the baby. Of the provider units in the survey, 44% reported carrying out some form of testing. In some units infection control staff had been involved initially, but when no growth of any organism was identified, regular testing was discontinued. Testing for infection involves resources in terms of time, money and disruption to the management of labour and birth, particularly if a number of samples and swabs are being taken. Recommendations on testing for infection vary and appear to be dependent on the experience of the authors of papers rather than being based on any evidence; there is a need to address this, particularly as related to infection transmitted through blood or body secretions.

Monitoring of progress in labour. Concerns exist about what constitutes adequate monitoring of the fetus underwater, particularly as the physiology of those babies who may be compromised and are subsequently born into water is unknown (Royal College of Obstetricians and Gynaecologists 1993). Electronic monitoring devices which can be used underwater are available and we found that 35% of units used these to monitor fetal well-being. Others used conventional Doppler machines with the transducer head protected by a condom or rubber glove. This protected transducer was then used underwater (with varying degrees of success) or more usually with the mother lifting her abdomen out of the water or standing up. It was unusual for women to be asked to leave the water except in some units where short periods of continuous cardiotocography were used prior to getting into the pool or at intervals in the labour.

For assessment of the progress in labour by vaginal examination, 38% of units said women were asked to leave the pool for this, 27% of units did not ask women to leave the water, carrying out the vaginal examination underwater, and 8% asked women to stand or kneel. The rest stated that the practice concerning vaginal examination varied depending on the mother and midwife involved.

Monitoring of maternal and fetal well-being is a contentious issue which remains unresolved in the care of women in normal labour out of water. The concern that a compromised fetus may breathe when being born into water adds another dimension to the argument which is not easily resolved without further research involving large clinical trials.

Analgesia in a birthing pool. One of the main benefits of using water in labour is the potential it has to provide non–pharmacological pain relief for women. This benefit is difficult to separate out from other effects of water immersion and to some extent the whole philosophy of care which surrounds the use of water, especially in a designated environment such as a birthing pool. Specific pain-relieving effects which are attributed to the use of immersion in water remain untested. The NPEU survey showed that other methods of pain relief were used when women were in the pool. It was uncommon for women to have pethidine and then enter the water, and a time period of at least 4 hours was quoted between administration of pethidine and entering the pool. The most common additional form of pain relief was the use of Entonox (nitrous oxide and oxygen; 92%). Of the 102 provider units (who used a birthing pool for more than four births), 39% offered other non-pharmacological methods of pain relief and relaxation such as aromatherapy and massage. Women's satisfaction with birthing pools tends to be high (E Burns 1995, pers. comm.) and a number of comparison studies show that women in a birthing pool use less additional pain relief (Burns & Greenish 1993, Garland & Jones 1994). It is still not possible, however, to deduce from this that it is the use of the water which provides the relief from pain. The reduction in the use of alternative analgesic agents could be related to other factors: for example, it could be that additional pain relief is less readily offered; that there is a benefit from the more constant supervision by the midwife when a woman is labouring in water; and the environment itself may have an influence on the woman's tolerance and perception of pain. Where additional agents for pain relief are used (as well as immersion in water), such as Entonox, this makes the specific pain-relieving effects of immersion in water very difficult to assess.

Birth in a pool

There has been a considerable growth in the number of births in water. The NPEU survey identified 1808 births in water in 1992, increasing to 2885 in 1993 within the NHS (Alderdice et al 1995a). In the NPEU study, six baby deaths were reported to us following birth in water for the 2-year period 1992–1993. It should be highlighted that reports of problems were likely to be incomplete because of our reliance on local data which were often not collected systematically. The full details of each case were not known, however in none of the cases was the outcome attributed to the birth taking place in water.

Deaths have been documented in other countries (Ward 1993, Zimmerman et al 1993). The death of a baby in Sweden in 1993 was felt to be a particular cause for concern as the post-mortem results suggested that the baby had inhaled contaminated water (Robinson 1993, Rosser 1994).

As discussed earlier in the chapter, in uncomplicated labour babies have an inhibitory reflex which reduces the likelihood of them gasping until exposed to an appropriate stimulus such as air. However the case reported in Sweden and also a case reported in the *British Medical Journal* describing a diagnosis of freshwater drowning (in a baby who made a full recovery) suggest that the physiology surrounding birth in water can no longer be considered as straightforward as it once was (Barry 1995). Much more research into the physiological issues is urgently needed.

Using a conventional bath

As already discussed there is a considerable difference in the advice offered and the use in practice of a conventional bath for labour and/or births in comparison to designated birthing pool use. This was highlighted in the NPEU survey when we asked respondents to describe their general practice when a conventional bath was used. We prompted on three key areas: temperature recommendation, fetal monitoring and other pain relief.

Women who used a conventional bath were reported to have intermittent routine monitoring while in the bath in 49% of hospitals providing this as a care option. A total of 38% of hospitals said they had temperature recommendations, with 18% using the same recommendations as they did for a birthing pool. Thirty-three percent said that analgesia, mainly Entonox, was offered when the mother was in the bath. Many commented that once other forms of pain relief were required the woman was asked to get out of the bath.

Advice to women using a bath at home, either before coming into hospital or when having a home delivery, tended to be very general, for example 'have a warm bath, not too hot'.

Routine births in a conventional bath were rare. Four provider units reported regularly using a conventional bath in hospital and five reported the use of conventional baths for birth at home. A number of other units reported births in a conventional bath, however these incidents were described as unplanned occurrences.

LABOUR AND BIRTH IN WATER: ONE HOSPITAL'S EXPERIENCE

A birthing pool was installed at the Women's Centre, John Radcliffe Hospital, Oxford in 1990 (see Fig. 9.1). Since then it has become part of a range of options for women in labour and has proved popular with approximately 5% of women opting to use the pool for labour and/or birth per year.

The use of water as an alternative to pharmacological pain relief in labour is greatly encouraged at the Women's Centre in Oxford. The birthing pool is in constant use and for those times when it is not available or those occasions when a woman might be advised against labouring in the pool, a shower is another available option and is recommended for some women in labour. Many women have found that water from a shower hose directed towards their lower back is very helpful during labour.

The pool is permanently installed in one of the delivery rooms. It is a cream-coloured, ovoid, non-slip pool positioned away from the walls to give all-round access. Water flows into the pool through eyelets in the side and the temperature of the water is thermostatically controlled. It takes approximately 10 minutes to fill and it empties rapidly through straight, wide drainage pipes. The cleaning protocol was drafted by the regional infection control officer and involves first rinsing the pool and then cleaning it using sanitising powder and rinsing this away. It is then dried thoroughly.

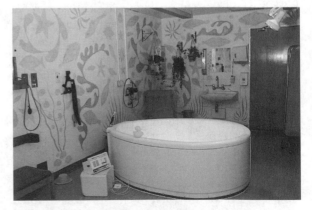

Figure 9.1 A typical water-birth room.

For women who wish to use the birthing pool, some assessment is made of their condition and progress in the pregnancy based on the following criteria: an uncomplicated pregnancy of 37 weeks or more gestation; a spontaneous onset of labour; being in established labour; and a cervix which is dilating.

First stage

The pool room is decorated with an aqua and terracotta seascape mural. The emphasis is on comfort and privacy for the woman. The lights are dimmed in preparation for use. The pool is filled at least up to the level of the mother's breasts when sitting in the pool but below the level of the water inlets. The water temperature is recorded and checked using a digital thermometer. The temperature of the water is recorded when the woman enters the pool; the temperature is then recorded when the woman enters the second stage and at the end of the third stage. In response to the concerns identified by practitioners in Bristol (Rosevear et al 1993), although no set temperature is prescribed the water is kept at a temperature which is comfortable for the woman but which is unlikely to exceed 38°C.

Maternal and fetal observations are carried out as they would be for a normal labour on dry land. Maternal observations are recorded on the partogram throughout all stages of labour. Vaginal examinations are performed when and if required in the water, or on dry land if the mother is out of the pool. Fetal monitoring is carried out with the use of a Sonicaid Dopplertone adapted for underwater use (Fig. 9.2). The pool water is kept as free as possible from contaminants such as faecal matter and blood clots by using a sieve to remove these when necessary.

Where a woman feels the need for additional pain relief, nitrous oxide and oxygen gas (Entonox) is offered for use in the pool, and lavender or chamomile oil may be added to the water if the woman wishes. Apart from these no other form of pain relief is offered while the woman is in the pool.

Second stage

During the second stage the woman pushes as and when she wishes. Traditional control of the head during crowning is not considered necessary and it is recommended that the midwife needs to give only verbal guidance to the mother at this point (Fig. 9.3 shows a mother and baby just after birth in water; Fig. 9.4 show the same baby just after birth).

Where there is concern about the progress of labour or of the birth, there are two options available to the care-givers. In the case of a problem in the labour and probable need for intervention, the mother will need to be helped out of the pool. In the case of problems arising during the actual delivery, such as shoulder dystocia, the mother may not need to leave the pool but the water needs to be emptied immediately and then the

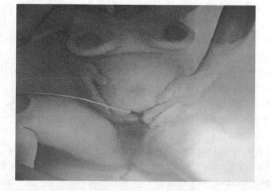

Figure 9.2 A woman being monitored during labour in a birthing pool.

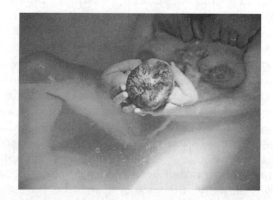

Figure 9.3 Mother and baby immediately after birth in a pool.

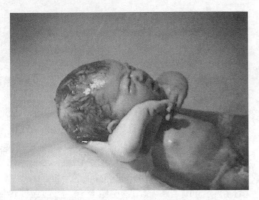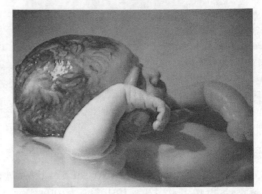

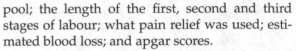
Figure 9.4 Baby immediately after birth in a pool.

emergency can be dealt with in a similar way as if it had occurred on dry land.

Third stage

If all is well following delivery, a physiological third stage can be managed without getting the woman out of the pool. The placenta is then delivered underwater. The mother holds the baby with the head above the water and the rest of the body at the level of her uterus. The cord remains unclamped. If blood loss appears excessive the mother is helped out of the pool and appropriate action taken. Postnatal observations are completed in the usual way.

Postnatal evaluation

A pool evaluation form is completed by the midwife and mother. Auditing of birthing pool use has been in place since 1990 when it was first used. As a consequence, a very extensive database is now available. An analysis of the use of water from August 1990 to October 1993 showed that a total of 1067 women used the pool during that time. Of these women, 604 (57%) were primiparas and 463 (43%) multiparas. The average age was 29 (SD = 5.6). A total of 389 women (36%) used the pool for labour only and 678 (64%) gave birth in water. A number of outcome variables have been recorded since 1990: state of perineum after delivery; the mother's and the partner's opinion of the pool; the midwife's opinion of the

pool; the length of the first, second and third stages of labour; what pain relief was used; estimated blood loss; and apgar scores.

The evaluation forms, guidelines and clinical practice continue to evolve as new research findings emerge, as midwives identify concerns and develop new innovations. For example, the introduction of the digital thermometer led to a change in how the temperature was recorded and details of temperature were therefore added to the evaluation form. As so much information has been computerised on the auditing of the pool use, work is presently underway to find appropriate retrospective controls for a comparison study.

THE WAY AHEAD

The choice to labour in water appears to have been adopted alongside conventional options in the current provision of maternity care. How long it will maintain this support can only be subject to conjecture. Birthing pools, particularly portable ones, have been open to criticism. One self-employed midwife commented in the NPEU survey: 'The focus is on the pool rather than the mother. Fiddling with buckets, hoses around the pool ... The pool is so big it gets in the way, in small houses it is oppressive. Pools can dominate and control labour by their presence.'

As hospitals are being built, or existing maternity facilities renovated, provider units are integrating rooms with large baths or birthing pools into their building proposals. Even if birth in water becomes a rare event, a woman labouring in water will still have the space and buoyancy that large baths and birthing pools allow.

If the trend towards the increasing use of water for labour and birth continues, this may pose more of a challenge to already stretched health service resources. More midwives are required, a midwife needs to be in constant attendance with a woman in a birthing pool, and two midwives are usually present for the birth. In offering something which is only available on a limited basis, there is the possibility that some women may feel disappointed or let down by the service if it transpires that the birthing pool is not available for them after their expectations have been raised.

If it is felt that it is the use of warm water that is beneficial rather than the size of container the labour takes place in, then it may be important to discuss this with women in the antenatal period. This might lead to more choices for labour—for example, labouring in a conventional sized bath or using a shower may also prove beneficial. As specially designed and marketed pools have emerged, the use of conventional baths and showers appears to have taken a back seat, and this is reflected, at least in part, in the lack of formality in how they are used and in how that use is subsequently recorded.

As more research becomes available, the practice should continue to evolve. Auditing the use of water for all occasions is important, not only to examine the outcomes of practice but also to influence future practice.

SUMMARY

The use of immersion in water for pain relief in labour has become available to more women over the past couple of years and is popular with those who have experience of it, both women and caregivers alike. If evidence becomes available to support the formal use of birthing pools then changes in practice will be required to ensure that these are used in safe and effective ways.

As conventional baths and showers are widely used in health service care, it is important that as much attention is paid to advice and practice with these as is paid to the use of a birthing pool. The NPEU survey identified considerable discrepancies between the reported practices associated with the use of conventional baths and those associated with the use of birthing pools, even when the birthing pool was used for labour only. Although conventional bath use is largely informal and seen to be part of normal practice, many practice issues discussed in relation to the birthing pool have implications for the conventional bath, not only in terms of possible benefits but also in terms of risks. For example, if there are risks caused by temperature and infection in birthing pools, surely women who use conventional baths may be exposed to these risks too?

At this time the effect of immersion in water on pain perception in labour remains unclear. There is a need for large studies, particularly randomised controlled trials, to adequately assess pain relief and other possible effects surrounding the use of immersion in water.

Concerns about the effects of temperature and the possibility of a baby breathing when being born into water need to be addressed urgently by carrying out physiological research. More attention also needs to be paid to the reporting of problems. Researchers from the Institute of Child Health, through the British Paediatric Association Surveillance Unit, are monitoring adverse outcomes, including deaths, for babies whose mothers laboured and/or gave birth in water, and their research will give a more accurate description of any problems. To aid such research more widespread detailed auditing is required where immersion in water is routinely used.

As a method of non-pharmacological pain relief, the use of immersion in water in labour might be a desirable and effective option for both the mother and the baby. However the potential of immersion in water in terms of benefits or harm is still unknown. The more established its use becomes in the absence of substantive research, the harder it will be to assess, and the reality of women being able to exercise their informed choice of this as an option for labour or for birth will become more unlikely.

REFERENCES

Alderdice F A, Renfrew M J, Marchant S, Ashurst H, Hughes P, Berridge G, Garcia J 1995a Labour and birth in water in England and Wales. British Medical Journal 310 (6983): 837

Alderdice F A, Renfrew M J, Marchant S, Ashurst H, Hughes P, Berridge G, Garcia J 1995b Labour and birth in water in England and Wales: survey report. British Journal of Midwifery 3 (7): 375–382

Balaskas J, Gordon Y 1992 Waterbirths. Thorsons, London

Barry C 1995 Waterbirths: could saline in the pool reduce the potential hazards? British Medical Journal 310 (6994): 1602

Bastide A 1992 A randomized controlled trial of the effects of a whirlpool bath on labour, birth and the postpartum. Unpublished trial. Oxford Database of Perinatal Trials; Disk issue 8 (version 1.2): Record 5789

Burns E, Greenish K 1993 Pooling information: immersion in water during labour and delivery is an innovation in midwifery care but little research is available. Nursing Times 89 (8): 47–49

Cammu H, Clasen K, Van Wettere L 1992 Is having a warm bath during labour useful? Journal of Perinatal Medicine 20 (1): 104

Cammu H, Clasen K, Van Wettere L, Derde M 1994 'To bathe or not to bathe' during the first stage of labor. Acta Obstetricia et Gynecologica Scandinavica 73 (6): 468–472

Church L K 1989 Water birth: one birthing center's observations. Journal of Nursing and Midwifery 34 (4): 165–170

Department of Health 1993 Changing childbirth. Part 1: report of the Expert Maternity Group, part 2: survey of good communications practice in maternity services. HMSO, London

Doniec-Ulman I, Kokot F, Wambach G, Drab M 1987 Water immersion-induced endocrine alterations in women with EPH gestosis. Clinical Nephrology 28 (2): 51–55

Garland D, Jones K 1994 Waterbirth, 'first-stage' immersion or non-immersion? British Journal of Midwifery 2 (3): 113–120

Harmsworth G 1994 Safety first. Nursing Times 90 (11): 30–32

Hawkins S 1995 Water vs conventional births: infection rates compared. Nursing Times 91 (11): 38–40

Leboyer F 1991 Birth without violence. Mandarin, London

Lederman R P, Lederman E, Work B A, McCann D S 1978 The relationship of maternal anxiety, plasma catecholamines, and plasma cortisol to progress in labor. American Journal of Obstetrics and Gynecology 132: 495–500

Lenstrup C, Schantz A, Berget A, Feder E, Roseno H, Hertel J 1987 Warm tub bath during delivery. Acta Obstetricia et Gynecologica Scandinavica 66: 709–712

Lines M 1993 Waterbirth: feedback from mothers and midwives. British Journal of Midwifery; 1 (6): 264–268

National Childbirth Trust 1995 Labour and birth in water. NCT, London

Nightingale C 1994 Water birth in practice. Modern Midwife 4 (1): 15–19

Odent M 1983 Birth under water. Lancet ii: 1476–1477

Rawal J, Shah A, Stirk F, Mehtar S 1994 Waterbirth and infection in babies. British Medical Journal 309 (6953): 511

Reid T 1994 Water work. Nursing Times 90 (11): 26–30

Robinson J 1993 A waterbirth death in Sweden. AIMS Journal 5 (3): 7–8

Rosenthal M J 1991 Warm-water immersion in labor and birth. Female Patient 16: 35–46

Rosevear S K, Fox R, Stirrat G M 1993 Birthing pools and the fetus. Lancet 342 (8878): 1048–1049

Rosser J 1994 Is water birth safe? The facts behind the controversy. MIDIRS Midwifery Digest 4 (1): 4–6

Royal College of Obstetricians and Gynaecologists 1993 Statement on birth underwater. Press release, October 15

Royal College of Midwives 1994 The use of water during birth: position statement. RCM, London

Rush J 1992 Trial to assess the effects of the availability of a whirlpool bath for women in labour on the use of pharmacological pain relief, dystocia and the use of oxytocin for augmentation of labour. Ongoing trial. Oxford Database of Perinatal Trials, disk issue 8 (version 1.2): record 6382

Rydhstrom H 1992 Trial to test the effect of bathing vs no bathing in labour on transfer to neonatal intensive care. Ongoing trial. Oxford Database of Perinatal Trials, disk issue 8 (version 1.2): record 7199

Scheller M, Terinde R 1994 [An accident during a relaxation bath]. Zeitschrift fur Geburtshilfe und Perinatologie 198 : 104–105

Schorn M N, McAllister J L, Blanco J D 1993 Water immersion and the effect on labour. Journal of Nursing and Midwifery 38 (6): 336–342

Sidenblah E 1993 Waterbabies: Igor Tjarkovsky and his method of delivering and training children in water. A & C Black, London

Simpkin P 1989 Non-pharmacological methods of pain relief during labour. In: Chalmers I, Enkin M, Keirse M J N C (eds) Effective care in pregnancy and childbirth. OUP, Oxford, pp 813–912

Waldenstrom U 1994 Warm tub bath and sauna in early pregnancy: risk of malformation uncertain. Acta Obstetricia et Gynecologica Scandinavica 73 (6): 449–451

Waldenstrom U, Nilsson C 1992 Warm tub bath after spontaneous rupture of the membranes. Birth 19 (2): 57–63

Walker J 1994 Birth underwater: sink or swim. British Journal of Obstetrics and Gynaecology 101 (6): 467–468

Ward D 1993 Baby's death raises pool birth concern. The Guardian, October 16

Zimmerman R, Huch A, Huch R 1993 Water birth–is it safe? Journal of Perinatal Medicine 21 (1): 5–11

10

Transcutaneous electrical nerve stimulation

Rosalind Davies

LEARNING OUTCOMES

At the end of this chapter the reader will have

- **an increased awareness of the historical context of transcutaneous nerve stimulation (TENS)**

- **an introduction to the evidence surrounding the use of TENS in labour**

- **an introduction to a study undertaken into the effectiveness of TENS in labour**

- **an understanding of the use and application of TENS**

- **considered some of the potential contraindications for the use of TENS**

- **identified the roles of the midwife and the obstetric physiotherapist in the management of TENS for pain relief**

- **access to manufacturers and suppliers of TENS units.**

Transcutaneous electrical nerve stimulation (TENS) is the transmission of electrical energy across the surface of the skin via surface electrodes to the nervous system.

A HISTORICAL REVIEW

The effects and benefits produced by applying electrical energy to the human body has fascinated and intrigued mankind throughout the ages. It is believed that ancient civilisations such as the Egyptians used electrical energy produced from natural sources in the environment to alleviate painful conditions. The first reported use of electrical energy for pain relief was noted by a Roman physician by the name of Scribonius Largus in the year AD 46. He prescribed the use of electrogenic torpedo fish capable of generating electric shocks of 100–150 volts for the treatment of headaches and gout (Kane & Taub 1975, Miller Jones 1980, Hymes 1984). It was believed that when placed under the feet, the electrical charge from a torpedo fish cured arthritis, and even haemorrhoids were believed to have been successfully treated.

Following the classification and generalisation of the phenomenon of electricity by William Gilbert (1544–1603), many electrical generators and apparatus were produced which were capable of storing electrical energy. The first English language book on medical electricity was written by Richard Lovatt in 1756. It was called *Subtle medium proved* and listed cures for many painful complaints. Fascinated by the therapeutic effects of electrical energy John Wesley, the Methodist church leader, became a clinician. In 1759 he published *Electricity made plain and useful by a lover of mankind and of common sense*. Sciatica, headache, gout, Raynaud's phenomenon, pleuritic pain and angina pectoris were all conditions noted to be relieved by electrical energy (Hymes 1984). The forerunner of the electrical capacitor was the Heydon jar which was invented in 1745. It provided the capability of storing electrical energy and conserving quantities of charge for later use. Hospitals at this time were beginning to be equipped with electrotherapy equipment. In 1767 a new 'electrical shock machine' was installed in the Middlesex Hospital, London. Throughout the eighteenth and nineteenth centuries a multitude of investigators continued to use electrical energy to relieve many painful conditions. Rockwell et al (1875) produced a book which summarised the guidelines for competency required by physicians using electrotherapy along with application procedures and indications for its use.

In the twentieth century with the introduction of non-steroidal anti-inflammatory drugs (NSAIDs) and other efficient analgesia, the use of electrotherapy became rare in spite of its use in earlier ages. However, research work by neurophysiologists during the 1950s and 1960s (Hagbarth & Derr 1954, Collins & Randt 1958, Poggio & Mountcastle 1960, Shealy 1966, Wall 1967) provided relevant information for Melzack & Wall (1965) to propose their original 'gate-control theory'. Readers should refer to Chapter 3 for a further outline of this theory. The gate-control theory highlights the active role of the dorsal horn of the spinal cord in modulating sensory transmission. It suggests that stimulation in the large myelinated fibres (A fibres) will work through inhibitory circuits in the superficial laminae of the substantia gelatinosa of the dorsal horn to inhibit the transmission of activity in the small unmyelinated fibres (C fibres). The inhibitory circuits will act as a gate to nociceptive impulses. When C fibre transmission is greater than A fibre transmission the gate is opened and pain is perceived. If A fibre transmission can be increased, the gate is closed, leading to reduced or complete pain relief. Large diameter nerves can be stimulated at low current intensities and have been found to transmit impulses at high frequencies. Therefore low intensity, high frequency (100–200 Hz) TENS is appropriate and effective, and has been shown to stimulate A fibres (Janko & Trontelj 1980). TENS can therefore be assumed to produce pain relief through the mechanism proposed by Melzack & Wall. It should be noted that there has been some criticism of the theory which has been subsequently modified (Nathan 1976); however, the main aspect of the theory has been verified electrophysiologically, behaviourally and clinically (Woolf 1994).

Shealy (1966), a prominent neurophysiologist, considered that direct stimulation of the dorsal column of the spinal cord could inhibit the transmission of pain to higher pain perception centres in the brain. Shealy (1973, 1974) and Long (1974a, b) both evaluated patients for dorsal column electrode implantation by initially using transcutaneous nerve stimulation. TENS was noted by many patients to reduce pain almost as well as dorsal column implants. TENS subsequently became an important therapy in pain clinics.

The intensity, or strength, of an electrical current or stimulus is measured in milliamperes (mA) or volts (V). The frequency of the electrical pulses, which is measured in hertz (Hz), is defined as the number of pulses per second, pulse rate or the pulse frequency.

All electrical currents (pulses) which stimulate nerve tissue (excluding implanted stimulators) are transcutaneous electrical nerve stimulations. However, the term TENS is normally only given to stimulations produced by battery-operated, low intensity sensory nerve stimulators used for pain control. The electrical pulses produced by TENS units are of a variety of pulse widths, frequencies and intensities. The majority of TENS units produce what are termed 'symmetrical' or 'asymmetrical bi-phasic pulses' (see Figs 10.1 and 10.2). The pulse durations are often fixed. The duration, or pulse width, can, however, be from 0.02 up to 0.4 milliseconds (ms); see examples shown in Figure 10.3. The train of packets or pulses need not necessarily be constant but can take several forms, as follows (see Fig. 10.4):

- short trains of high frequency pulses produced at low intensity
- long trains of low frequency pulses at relatively high intensity
- short trains of high frequency and high intensity pulses.

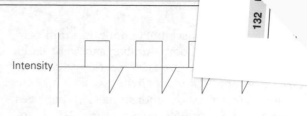

Figure 10.3   Variable width pulses.

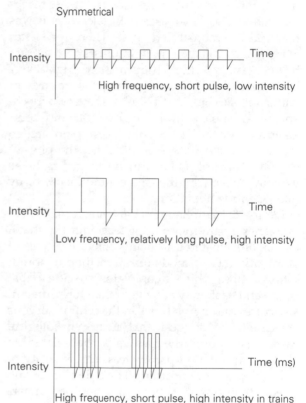

Symmetrical

High frequency, short pulse, low intensity

Low frequency, relatively long pulse, high intensity

High frequency, short pulse, high intensity in trains

Figure 10.4   Variations in pulse frequency, width and intensity.

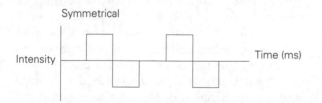

Figure 10.1   Symmetrical bi-phasic pulses.

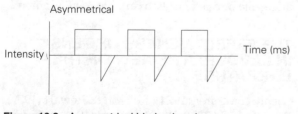

Figure 10.2   Asymmetrical bi-phasic pulses.

The frequency in most TENS units is variable. The ranges can be from 0 to 200 Hz. Voltage can be varied but will be limited to a relatively low intensity with the maximum current being 100 mA.

TENS has also been shown to relieve pain by increasing levels of endorphins (Salar et al 1981). Salar et al demonstrated that TENS, when applied for a period of 40 minutes at a frequency of 40–60 Hz continuously, and at a high intensity

40–80 mA, releases beta-endorphin into cere-brospinal fluid at both lumbar and ventricular sites. These experiments were carried out on people without chronic pain.

The discovery of morphine-like peptides, known as endorphins, occurred in 1975. It followed the discovery of opiate receptors, which are distributed widely throughout the central nervous system. When released, endorphins travel, and attach themselves, to the opiate receptors. This action increases pain tolerance. It was therefore demonstrated that TENS produces analgesia by blocking pain impulses to the brain by increasing A fibre transmission (Melzack & Wall 1965) and by stimulating the release of endorphins (Sjolund et al 1977). These two mechanisms are a basis from which to start in understanding how TENS produces pain relief. Readers should note, however, that the physiological action of TENS can no longer truly be explained solely by the gate-control theory or by neuropeptide liberation.

Lampe & Mannheimer (1984) noted that TENS is a general pain-modulating technique but that it can be administered in many different modes of stimulation. Each mode uses a method of stimulation pattern which is completely specific to that mode and each may activate completely different structures and nerve fibres in the central nervous system. They suggest that neurophysiological mechanisms and theories must be related to specific stimulation parameters. The majority of research papers concerning TENS do not contain adequate information on stimulation parameters and electrode placement sites used. Clarification regarding stimulation parameters must therefore be addressed in future studies. Thompson (1988), in a review of the pharmacology of stimulation analgesia, with particular respect to TENS, wrote that direct and indirect evidence suggests that monoamines such as 5-hydroxytryptamine (5HT or serotonin), noradrenaline (Nad), amino acids such as gamma aminobutyric acid (GABA), and opioid peptides (beta-endorphin and enkephalins), may all be involved. The neuropharmacological response to TENS appears to depend mainly on frequency and intensity of stimulation. Low frequency (2–10 Hz)/high intensity stimulation activates opioid systems, whereas high frequency (50–100+ Hz)/low intensity stimulation activates non-opioid systems.

Melzack & Wall (1982), using the McGill Pain Questionnaire, measured and recorded labour as producing one of the most severe forms of pain. Crawford (1984) suggested that pain relief poses a major problem in labour and that the present methods of analgesia appear to meet the needs of most parturients but are not without contraindications and complications. Throughout the 1970s and early 1980s improvements and developments were required, particularly in the area of producing a form of pain relief that could be self-administered, non-invasive, that was effective, and which would interfere minimally with the possibilities of a spontaneous natural vaginal delivery as well as enabling mobility and positions for comfort. I was very interested in the value of TENS for acute and chronic pain conditions. Together with Mr S. Crawford, Consultant Anaesthetist at Birmingham Maternity Hospital (now known as Birmingham Women's NHS Health Care Trust) at this time, we discussed the value of TENS for pain relief in labour. Although I felt that there was research available which already demonstrated its effectiveness for pain relief, as an obstetric physiotherapist, I was encouraged to evaluate its use during labour for women at the Birmingham Maternity Hospital during 1986. The results supported findings of previous research. Following the presentation of my findings, TENS units were purchased and TENS was made available to women in labour as a standard method of pain relief. I continued to develop talks about TENS and provided demonstrations for women booked for delivery at the hospital; a training programme for the midwifery staff was also developed. Following the study, TENS is now regarded as an important form of analgesia and is readily available to all women.

THE EFFECTIVENESS OF TENS IN LABOUR: A REVIEW OF THE LITERATURE

Shealy & Maurer (1974), Robson & Stewart (1979), Erkkola et al (1980), Bundsen et al (1981), Bundsen

& Ericson (1982) and Tawfik et al (1982) have all indicated that TENS was safe and effective to use in labour. Erkkola et al (1980) conducted a trial which involved 200 women. Of 100 women who used TENS, 31% reported good pain relief and 55% reported moderate pain relief. Bundsen et al (1981) found that TENS reduced pain in the first stage of labour, but that suprapubic pain was not relieved for the majority of these women. Tawfik et al (1982) noted that of 35 primigravidae using TENS, 14% recorded having excellent pain relief, 29% good pain relief and 57% satisfactory relief. Augustinsson et al (1977) reported that out of 147 patients using TENS in labour, 48% obtained good to very good pain control, 37% obtained moderate relief and the remainder had no benefit. German studies support and confirm significantly good results without any complications or side-effects on either the fetus or the mother (Kubista et al 1978, Neumark et al 1978).

Bundsen et al (1982) reported that there were no ill effects produced in the newborn infant when TENS is used by the mother. This had been previously noted in Bundsen et al (1981).

Birmingham Maternity Hospital study (Davies 1989)

The aim of this study, which involved 50 women, was to verify previous findings that TENS is an effective method of pain relief in labour. The limitations of this study, particularly methodological problems of conducting research on self-selecting groups, and the small sample size, are acknowledged. However, it is anticipated that other professionals will be encouraged to undertake further research in this area of pain relief in labour.

Background and method

The TENS equipment used for the study were two Spembly Obstetric Pulsar Units, which produce bi-phasic pulses. These were variable in amplitude and frequency, as follows—amplitude: 0.48 mA into 1 kohm load; frequency, normal mode: 15-200 Hz modulated at 2 bursts/sec, 180 msec on, 320 msec off; boost (continuous mode): 15–200 Hz, pulse width = 200 sec fixed.

The TENS machines were powered by 9 V batteries. The electrodes were standard carbon rubber (re-usable), and the contact medium was electrode gel. Adhesive strapping was used to fix and maintain electrodes over the appropriate nerve roots, making it possible for the women to move freely and to be able to adopt whatever positions would be comfortable throughout labour. Care was taken not to cover the electrode/lead junction in case the leads became detached. The electrodes were re-gelled every 4 hours to prevent drying out which could have reduced the effectiveness of the stimulation. It is important to note that, with use, impedance increases with this type of electrode and they should therefore be replaced at intervals.

Electrodes were positioned parallel with the woman's spine, the top pair of electrodes extending from T10 to L1, and the lower pair of electrodes between S2 and S4. These levels were chosen because nociceptive impulses from the body of the uterus and cervix are transmitted through T10, T11, T12 and L1 nerve roots. Nociceptive impulses from the perineal structures are transmitted by the pudendal nerve into the spinal cord, via the posterior roots of S2, S3 and S4. Nociceptive impulses from other pelvic structures involved in the pain of parturition, for example pelvic parietal peritoneum and uterine ligaments, are supplied by the lower lumbar and upper sacral nerves. Abdominal electrodes were considered for use in the study, but research carried out by Bundsen et al (1981) concluded that although fetal heart irregularities were not reported when abdominal TENS electrodes were used, there was a theoretical possibility that high intensity stimulation with conventional electrodes over the parturient's lower abdomen could, in unfavourable cases, induce irregularities of the fetal heart function (Bundsen & Ericson 1982). TENS may occasionally cause interference on a cardiotocograph used to record the fetal heart. Although this is more likely to occur if a fetal scalp transducer is in use for electronic fetal heart rate monitoring, it does not normally occur if an external transducer is being used.

In initial studies the electrodes positioned paravertebrally over the dermatomes of T10–L1 were used during the first stage of labour. For the second stage of labour the additional electrodes over the dermatomes S2–S4 were brought into use. More recent work has been done using all four positions together during both first and second stages of labour (Bundsen et al 1981, 1982). It was with this knowledge that the women in the trial used and stimulated all four electrode positions simultaneously.

Women who were at least 28 weeks pregnant and attending parent education sessions at the Birmingham Maternity Hospital were invited to a talk and demonstration of TENS. This included a brief history on the development of TENS, and a simple explanation of how TENS is thought to influence pain, and the correct positioning and appropriate time of application of electrodes, i.e. the latent or early active phase of labour, and at least 30 minutes before any augmentation of labour. Correct use of the TENS unit, setting an initial intensity level, and variation of the frequency and boosting when appropriate were also discussed, as well as combining pethidine and/or Entonox with TENS.

All of the women were encouraged to have the electrodes on their backs for several minutes and to appreciate the various frequency ranges once the initial intensity level had been set. The reaction of their skins to the stimulation was noted. Husbands/partners were encouraged to attend and they were advised not to alter the intensity or frequency channels of the TENS units for their partners when in labour. However, they could press the boost mode button at her request. A total of 50 women agreed to participate in the study. Midwives and midwifery students also attended the sessions to familiarise themselves with the function and application of TENS, as well as to acquire an appreciation of the sensation which TENS produces.

It has been suggested that there may be a link between beta-endorphin levels and neonatal respiratory depression. TENS has also been shown to produce these peptides (Salar et al 1981). It was therefore necessary to consider whether the combination of such deliveries with TENS could be a factor in producing higher concentration levels of beta-endorphins, thus requiring more frequent administration of naloxone. As such, it was important to record whether naloxone was administered to the infant following delivery.

It was also important to observe whether TENS interfered with the fetal monitoring in labour, particularly when a fetal scalp electrode (FSE) was used. If any interference was observed, medical staff were informed and a decision was then made as to whether TENS was maintained or discontinued.

Results

Group 1. All were normal deliveries, TENS being the only form of pain relief used.

Six out of the 50 women had a normal delivery and used only TENS throughout labour. Two of these women were primigravidae and four were multigravidae. The average length of labour was 6 hours. Four complained of back pain during labour and all six found TENS very beneficial in reducing pain. Two found that pain was completely relieved.

Figure 10.5 shows the level of pain experienced by 29 women who suffered from back pain at the onset or during labour. The first scale records the

Degree of back pain before any form of pain relief

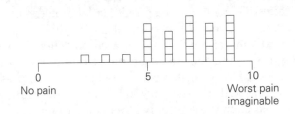

Degree of back pain when using TNS

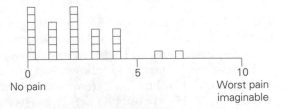

Figure 10.5 Level of back pain at the onset, or during labour, before and after TENS was applied (group 1).

pain without any form of pain relief and the second scale records the pain level once TENS was applied.

Although all four multiparae felt that their contractions were stronger during the current labour, TENS was extremely helpful in reducing pain intensity levels, particularly when boosted. Several found boosting very helpful when undergoing vaginal examination. One forgot to boost on several occasions during a contraction and noted the difference in relief of pain when she remembered. All the women in this group stated that they would use TENS again in labour. Two used TENS during suturing, but did not feel it was of any significant value at this time. Apgar scores recorded at delivery for all babies were within normal limits.

Group 2. All were normal deliveries; the women used TENS initially then combined it with pethidine or Entonox or both.

Figure 10.6 shows pain intensity levels before any form of pain relief was used, and then when

TENS was used initially, and finally when TENS was combined with pethidine or Entonox or both.

There were 15 women in this group, including a twin delivery: two used TENS initially, then combined it with pethidine; seven used TENS first then combined it with Entonox; and six used TENS initially, then combined it with both pethidine and Entonox. Eleven of the women were primigravidae and four were multigravidae. The average length of labour was 9 hours. Three of the 15 labours were induced. Ten complained of back pain. All 15 women found TENS to be very helpful in the early active phase of labour. As they progressed, all found combining it with pethidine or Entonox, or both, very successful. All would use TENS again. The TENS leads became detached during one woman's labour; when the leads were reapplied she was able to appreciate the effectiveness of TENS.

Possible interference with FSE monitoring was noted in two labours. For one of these, the level of interference was unacceptable in the presence of several low baseline fetal heart rate recordings. TENS was therefore discontinued.

One particular woman was very impressed with TENS which she used following a membrane sweep and insertion of a prostaglandin pessary. She had been unable to sleep due to discomfort but once she was given a TENS unit she was able to sleep, relaxed and free of 'prostin' pain.

All babies in this group had normal Apgar scores.

Group 3 (Fig. 10.7). All were forceps deliveries. Women used TENS initially, then combined it with pethidine or Entonox, or both.

There were eight women in this group: seven were primigravidae and one a multipara. One used only TENS until her baby was delivered by Simpson's forceps under a pudendal anaesthetic block. One woman with pre-eclampsia used TENS for 1 hour following induction of labour, but did not find it helpful. She discontinued using it. The remaining six women found it very helpful initially. One went on to combine it with pethidine and five found the combination of TENS, pethidine and Entonox more suitable. Five of these women had the TENS removed when pudendal blocks were administered. The sixth

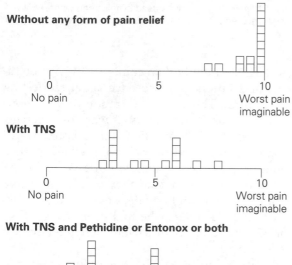

Without any form of pain relief

With TNS

With TNS and Pethidine or Entonox or both

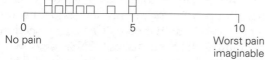

Figure 10.6 Level of pain experienced by the women in group 2 during labour before any form of pain relief was used; then when TENS was used initially; and when TENS was combined with pethidine or Entonox, or both.

Without any form of pain relief

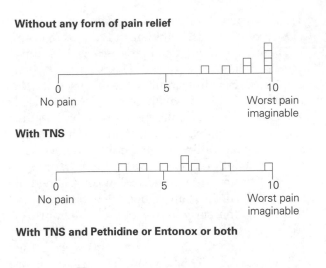

With TNS

With TNS and Pethidine or Entonox or both

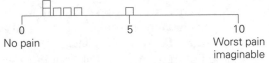

Figure 10.7   Level of pain experienced by the women in group 3 during labour before any form of pain relief was used; then when TENS was used initially; and when TENS was combined with pethidine or Entonox, or both.

Without any form of pain relief

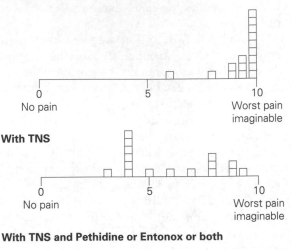

With TNS

With TNS and Pethidine or Entonox or both

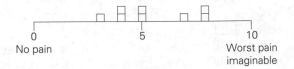

Figure 10.8   Level of pain experienced by the women in group 4 during labour before any form of pain relief was used; then when TENS was used initially; and when TENS was combined with pethidine or Entonox, or both.

woman in this group had the TENS unit removed because of unacceptable interference with the FSE recording in the presence of low baseline recordings. Naloxone was administered to this woman's baby. She had received 100 mg of pethidine 3 hours before delivery. TENS had been removed 2 hours before delivery. The average duration of labour was 13 hours. One of three women who complained of back pain obtained complete relief. Two of these women experienced labour with the baby in a persistent occipito-posterior position. Two found that TENS helped to relieve their labour pain considerably. All would use TENS again.

Group 4 (Fig. 10.8). All were delivered following use of epidural anaesthesia in labour, TENS being used initially.

There were 16 women in this group: fourteen were primigravidae and two were multigravidae. Eight women used TENS for 75% of the duration of their labours and then requested an epidural; six used TENS initially, then combined it with Entonox before requesting an epidural; and two

used TENS initially then combined it with pethidine and Entonox before once again requesting an epidural. The average duration of the labour was 16 hours. The epidural was, on average, requested after 75% duration of the labour. Twelve women complained of back pain, whereas three found it gave them complete relief. A total of 15 out of the 16 women said they would use TENS again. One woman had very slight skin soreness under the electrodes; she had been using TENS for 12 hours. All babies were delivered with a normal Apgar score.

Group 5 (Fig. 10.9). There were five women in this group, four primigravidae and one multipara. All were delivered by Caesarean section.

Initially, they all used TENS. One woman required a Caesarean section because of fetal distress. The remaining four then used Entonox with TENS. One woman in this group had a Caesarean section under general anaesthetic because of fetal

Without any form of pain relief

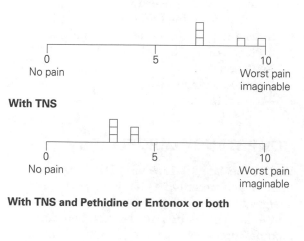

With TNS

With TNS and Pethidine or Entonox or both

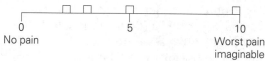

Figure 10.9 Level of pain experienced by the women in group 4 during labour before any form of pain relief was used; then when TENS was used initially; and when TENS was combined with pethidine or Entonox, or both.

distress following 13 hours of labour, during which time she was coping well with her contractions. The remaining three women requested epidural anaesthesia for their delivery. Only one woman in this group complained of back pain before using TENS. All of them would use TENS again.

Discussion

Although TENS can be applied at any stage of labour, it has been shown to be most helpful in the latent and early active phases of most labours. Johnson (1995, pers. comm.) has recently undertaken a survey evaluating women's views after use of TENS in labour. Over 10 000 women in the UK participated in the study. It was found that 7122 parturients (71%) reported excellent or good relief of pain by TENS, while 648 (6%) noted poor relief. A total of 8645 women (86%) received addi-

tional analgesics (pethidine, Entonox and epidurals) during labour. Of 14% completing labour without additional analgesia, 1187 (83%) reported excellent or good pain relief. It has been suggested that women who have short duration labours and are coping well with breathing techniques and positions of comfort may find it is all they need. Harrison et al (1987) suggest that women who used TENS alone also have shorter labours than when supplementary analgesia is needed; this was also noted by Nesheim (1981). On the other hand, Jones (1980) found no significant difference in the length of labours between those who used TENS and those who did not. TENS may be easily combined with pethidine and/or Entonox in labour to reduce the pain intensity of contractions. In prolonged labours, some women may be mobile for 75% of the time and then progress to an epidural without being left with any unwanted side-effects.

In the Birmingham study, TENS was found to be of value in relieving discomfort following intervention from procedures such as prostaglandin induction of labour, and backache prior to and during labour and vaginal examination. All the women commented on the distraction element of the stimulation and the importance of varying it during labour. One even used the boost mode whilst an intravenous infusion was being inserted into her arm.

Occasionally, interference was noted on the electronic cardiotocograph (CTG) recordings. However, this was not a major problem. It mainly occurred when the boost mode was used on the TENS apparatus. Harrison et al (1987) recorded no low Apgar scores, even though one baby in the study group required administration of naloxone; however, in this case, 100 mg of pethidine had been administered to the mother 3 hours before the delivery.

Women are now questioning the effects of various forms of pain relief both on themselves and their babies. The non-invasive nature of TENS is certainly an important factor for many women. In addition, TENS does not restrict mobility, another important factor. The ability to be in personal control of pain relief is often a major consideration for women in labour when using TENS. Partners will occasionally assist by boosting the stimulation at the command of the women. Throughout this study all birthing partners were instructed that it was important not to alter the intensity or frequency controls without direction from the woman.

In his survey, Johnson (1995, pers. comm.) identified that 9160 parturients (91%) said that they would use TENS again to manage labour pain. Harrison et al (1987) found that post-delivery comments of women and midwives showed TENS to give considerable consumer satisfaction, and the safety element of the method was confirmed. The current study found that 49 out of the 50 women would use TENS again.

The only known side-effect from use of TENS in the study was the slight skin irritation recorded by one woman. During the demonstration sessions only one woman showed slight irritation and reddening of the skin after only five minutes of stimulation. The causes of skin irritation will be discussed later. No other side-effect or complications were noted.

Possible placebo effect

Thorsteinsson et al (1977), in a double blind trial, found that TENS was more effective than placebo-TENS. A total of 48% of women in Thorsteinsson et al's study found TENS relieved labour pain and 32% obtained relief with placebo-TENS. Neumark et al (1978) found that TENS was more effective as an analgesic than was the placebo. Nesheim (1981), however, found no differences between TENS and TENS-placebo in degree of pain relief and further analgesia required. Harrison et al (1986) also found no significant differences between TENS and placebo-TENS with regard to pain relief. They did note that women using TENS and Entonox combinations required less additional analgesia. Consumer satisfaction was, however, much higher in the TENS group than in the placebo group.

Drugs that modify the effects of TENS analgesia

Thompson (1988) identified certain drugs which may be influenced when TENS is used:

- drugs with which the analgesic effect produced by TENS may be increased, e.g.
  —tryptophan
  —tricyclic antidepressants
  —D-phenylalanine (DPA)
- drugs that potentially decrease analgesia produced by TENS include
  —naloxone
  —benzodiazepines (Bz)
  —corticosteroids.

COMPETENCY GUIDELINES

Within the last 10–15 years TENS has become more widely accepted as having a part to play in analgesia during labour. Many maternity units now offer TENS for pain relief. There are now manufacturers who have produced obstetric TENS units in order to supply the demand by women to obtain a TENS unit which they can start using while at home, thus enabling them to commence use in early labour. There have been some TENS units which have been produced which are not suitable for the requirements of effective analgesia for labour pain.

Midwives have a professional responsibility to be aware of the physiological effects of TENS (as is understood at this point in time), the contraindications and precautions in its use and correct application procedures before undertaking application of TENS for a woman in labour.

The United Kingdom Central Council circular (UKCC 1991) states that:

… midwives may on their own responsibility manage pain relief in labour by the use of transcutaneous nerve stimulation provided that:

1. they have received adequate and appropriate instruction, which is a matter to be determined by agreed local policy, and

2. safety standards conform to those laid down by the Department of Health Medical Devices Directorate in England, or equivalent body in Scotland, Wales or Northern Ireland. The current standard for all medical equipment is set out in the British Standard specification BS 5724 Part 1 1989.

Midwives' attention must also be drawn to *The Midwives Code of Practice* (UKCC 1994), paragraphs

56 ('Complementary and alternative therapies') and 22 ('Responsibility for competency in new skills').

A proposal for a training programme for midwives

I have been involved in developing this training programme at Birmingham Maternity Hospital. It has been used and evaluated for some time. Midwives all have an interest in TENS and some attend a training programme to become trainers in order to pass on their knowledge and expertise to others. The training programme includes a brief history of and development of TENS, and an outline of the physiological explanations for modulation of pain using TENS. In addition, contraindications to its use, precautions required, and advice on methods of introducing and explaining TENS to women and their partners are included. The correct application of TENS is also an important part of the programme, as is the actual procedure for removal and cleaning of equipment.

It is part of local policy that each new trainer undertakes an oral, written and practical test of competency. The practical aspect involves applying the TENS unit to women attending the TENS talk and demonstration session, working closely with and utilising the knowledge and experience of the obstetric physiotherapist. The practical aspect of the 'examination' may be completed on the wards, in the delivery suite or in parent education sessions under supervision. Standards of competency can be maintained by regular refresher sessions with the obstetric physiotherapist. These trainers then undergo annual updating. This is particularly important in order to maintain and share knowledge of current research findings in relation to the use of TENS.

'TENS training manuals' have been developed to provide relevant information which is then available in all areas and departments. The obstetric physiotherapist and the midwives are thus able to work in cooperation and are available to offer constant advice and support to women at any time throughout pregnancy, labour or the immediate postnatal period.

OBSTETRIC TENS UNITS

An obstetric TENS unit is made up of an obstetric TENS machine, lead wires, electrodes and a battery. There are many obstetric TENS unit manufacturers, some of which are listed at the end of this chapter (see Fig. 10.10). It is in no way a comprehensive list and it is recommended that each manufacturer be contacted to obtain complete information regarding features and parameter specifications of their units. It should be noted that these TENS units may vary regarding intensity ranges produced. Some have been set at a fixed frequency and others have a fixed pulse width, while others have a variable pulse width facility. The controls also vary: some need to be continuously pressed during a contraction; others, once pressed at the start of a contraction, need only be released at the end. The Association of Physiotherapists in Women's Health (ACPOG; previously known as The Association of Chartered Physiotherapists in Obstetrics and Gynaecology) established a TENS Working Party which suggested criteria for the suitability of TENS equipment for use in labour (ACPOG 1992). An obstetric physiotherapist is therefore able to provide specific advice on particular facilities which may be important or useful in relation to any obstetric TENS unit. These criteria are incorporated in this text.

Contraindications of TENS

Contraindications, warnings and precautions should be included in the manufacturer's instruction manual or video and must be adhered to by women and midwives. Contraindications and precautions will include:

1. TENS must NOT be used by anyone who has a CARDIAC PACEMAKER. Ericksson et al (1978) suggest that TENS *could* be used by those individuals with an asynchronous, fixed rate pacemaker but was *not* to be used with demand-type cardiac pacemakers of synchronous type (ventricular inhibited, ventricular triggered and atrial synchronous). As most obstetric TENS unit manufacturers state that all cardiac pacemakers are contraindicated, it is important that this is *strictly adhered to*. Spembly Medical, who produce

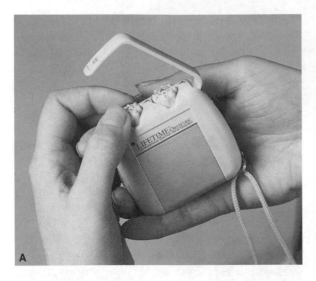

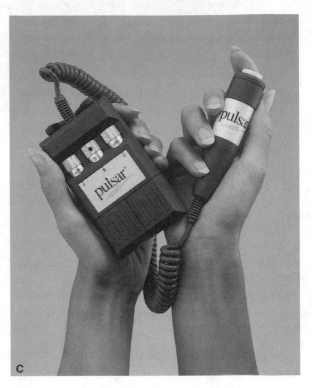

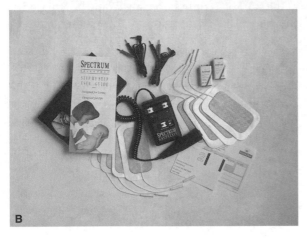

Figure 10.10 **A**. 'Lifetime Microtens' by Neen Health Care. **B**. 'SPECTRUM' by Promedics Ltd. **C**. 'Pulsar' by Spembly Medical. Addresses are given at the end of this chapter.

the Obstetric Pulsar Unit, specify that their unit must not be used by people with implanted cardiac demand type pacemakers.

2. TENS must NEVER be placed over the carotid sinus. Electrodes must not be placed on or around the area of the carotid sinus as this could lead to cardiac arrhythmias. Placement over the pharyngeal region could produce laryngeal and/or pharyngeal spasm interfering with blood pressure and respiration and leading to cardiac arrest.

3. TENS must NOT be used in the first trimester of pregnancy. Neen Management Systems state that their obstetric unit must not be used before the second trimester of pregnancy.

Promedics who produce the Spectrum obstetric TENS unit state that their unit must not be used before 37 weeks of pregnancy, unless under the specific guidance of a medical practitioner. Midwives who are competent in the use of TENS should only use it for analgesia for labour (from 37 weeks gestation).

Precautions

Care should be taken not to place the electrodes:

* over the eyes
* over superficial aspects of bone, such as the head and tibial shaft; the periosteum is highly innervated and thus very sensitive

- near the heart in people with cardiac problems
- over skin lesions or open cuts/wounds due to the risk of infection and varying resistance offered to the stimulation.

Midwives would not be placing electrodes in any of these positions but these precautions have been included so that women can be strongly advised to keep any hired TENS unit solely for their own use for labour and well out of the hands of playful and inquisitive children, or even adults. The following should also be adhered to:

- TENS should NOT be used by a woman if she is driving
- TENS should ONLY be used by women with epilepsy after full medical consultation
- TENS should NOT be continued should any skin irritation occur on the electrode sites; any such reaction should be investigated clinically.

Electrodes

For obstetric use the ideal size is 100 mm × 40 mm.

Re-usable carbon-silicone electrodes

These electrodes require tape, and gel or Karaya gum pads for adherence and activation respectively. Lampe & Mannheimer (1984) state that carbon-silicone electrodes should be replaced every 6 months even though no visible changes are apparent. The loss of electrical conductance of this electrode system over time will not be obvious but is always present. Some manufacturers advise that re-usable electrodes have an expected life of 12–18 months.

Cleaning after use

Wash electrodes in soapy warm water, then dry, clean with spirit and dry. (Local infection control policy may give advice on cleaning.) The leads need to be strong, flexible and particularly resistant to breakage. They are usually bifurcated into two. Some leads can be bifurcated into four; this enables the use of six electrodes with a dual channel unit. Again, there are some manufacturers who do not recommend using abdominal electrodes. Before use, leads must always be checked for any signs of wear and tear around the 'jack plug', termination pin, or the plastic casing of the actual lead. In such cases they must not be used and must not be covered over with tape, but replaced straight away with new leads.

Self-adhering disposable electrodes

These are attached to the skin by a hypoallergenic conductive gel. They are disposable after use. Manufacturers will state that they may be re-used by the same person for up to 15 times. If they become slightly detached during use, they can be reapplied by slightly moistening the surface of the gel with water.

Transmission gels

Hypoallergenic electrotransmission gels are produced by various obstetric TENS manufacturers. All appear to work well. Karaya gum pads can be used for women whose skin is very sensitive to creams, gels or rubber. Karaya is a naturally occurring conductive gum, which when moistened becomes adhesive. It should eliminate the need for electrode gel and fixing tape. When not being used the Karaya should be kept in a cool place. Water-soluble petroleum jelly should not be used as it is not an electrotransmissive medium.

Application to skin using tape

Re-usable electrodes need to be taped to the skin surface. It is essential that the tape is maintaining *complete* contact between the electrode and the skin. At times there may be a need to use a heavier form of taping than the more commonly used lightweight tapes. Never tape over the electrode–lead junction because, if the leads do become detached, this may then not be visible.

Battery

Battery-charger and batteries can be purchased from some obstetric TENS manufacturers. Ordinary batteries must not be used with such a battery charger.

APPLICATION OF TENS FOR RELIEF OF PAIN IN LABOUR

Care of the skin

Slight skin reactions at the electrode site are a rare occurrence. These may be due to the electrical current, composition of the electrodes, indequate conduction properties of the coupling gel, the adhesives used to fasten the electrodes in position, or, as is most likely, an inappropriate method of application for fastening the electrodes in position. Skin problems may therefore be due to:

* electrical causes
* chemical causes
* allergic causes
* mechanical causes.

Electrical causes. Skin burns may occur when excessive stimulation is used through electrodes of a small area. To ensure safety, the electrode surface area, as suggested by Lampe & Mannheimer (1984), should be equal to or greater than 4×4 cm. If the distance between the electrodes is less than the cross-sectional diameter of the electrodes, then the current density will be greater than that beneath either electrode. The heat produced may be sufficient to produce a skin burn. It is important to be aware that some manufacturers in their promotional advertisements position the electrodes too close together. Micropunctate burns (micropunctate areas being areas such as at hair follicles) may occur secondary to poor electrical contact between skin and the stimulating electrode. These burns could occur if re-usable electrodes are not gelled adequately or if the electrodes do not mould to the body contour. The current may concentrate around hair follicles, producing current densities within these small areas sufficiently high to produce a burn. Therefore, when using re-usable electrodes, the entire surface of the electrode should be completely covered with sufficient quantities of gel. The electrode must be re-gelled at least every 4 hours to avoid 'drying out'. An awareness of these errors of application will prevent skin complications.

Chemical causes. Chemical reactions within the skin structures are highly unlikely as causes of irritation. This is due to the fact that obstetric

TENS units produce bi-phasic pulses and so produce no net unbalanced ionic shift into the skin tissues and no acid–base concentrations. The units also generate pulses with very short durations.

Allergic causes. It is extremely rare that electrodes will cause an allergic reaction. It is only following very prolonged use of TENS over many treatment periods without the site of the electrodes being changed which could precipitate this very remote occurrence. This problem is therefore not normally of relevance for its relatively brief use in labour. There are some adhesive tapes which may cause skin reactions. Some electrode gels may contain chemicals or abrasive irritants that are present to improve electrical contact. It is suggested that skin reaction is probably not an allergic reaction but an irritant follicular reaction. Silicon oxide, as used in certain transmission gels, has in the past been considered to be an irritating substance. Hypoallergic electrotransmission gels are now produced by many obstetric TENS manufacturers.

Mechanical causes. Mechanical stresses may be produced by shearing forces between the tape and the skin. When attaching tape over electrodes, consider the flexion requirements for sitting, and for bending forwards within the thoracic and lumbar spines. It is important to tape electrodes individually to the skin and not to tape across a set of electrodes using one strip. If long strips of tape are placed parallel to the spinal columns, bending forward or sitting will produce very strong shearing stresses between skin and tape. Tape should be applied to the centre of the electrode first and then with sequential fastening from the centre towards one side and then towards the other.

Application of electrodes

Always clean and dry the skin before applying the electrodes. Do not position the electrodes over scars, moles or other skin blemishes.

For self-adhesive electrodes (disposable):

1. firmly connect leads to the electrodes
2. remove electrodes from backing sheet and apply one by one to appropriate sites

3. apply carefully and avoid hand contact with the adhesive side of the electrode
4. To ensure good contact press firmly down on to the electrode.

For re-usable electrodes:

1. firmly connect leads to the electrodes
2. apply sufficient electrode gel to the flat side of each electrode to cover the entire surface
3. apply to the skin pressing down firmly
4. fix securely in place with tape.

Electrode placement (see Fig. 10.11)

Top pair of electrodes. The top pair of electrodes must be positioned on either side of the spine between T10 and L2, where T10 represents the spine of the tenth thoracic vertebra and L2 represents the spine of the second lumbar vertebra. The upper limit of T10 may be found by firstly locating the tip of the inferior angle of the scapula; then by tracing an imaginary line from the tip of the inferior angle of the scapula towards the midline, until the spine of T7—the spine of the seventh thoracic vertebra—is located.

The spinous process of a vertebra feels like a very small slightly raised lump. When T7 has been located, palpate using fingertips down over the thoracic spinous processes of T8 and T9, to T10.

The top of each electrode must be placed at this level and *not* any higher. It must be noted that when someone is anxious, stressed or in pain,

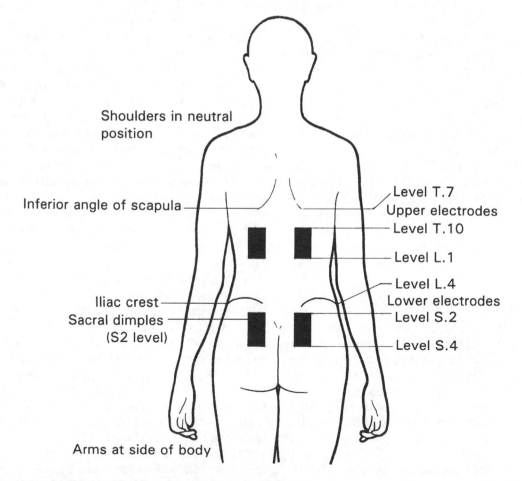

Figure 10.11   Positioning of TENS electrodes for use in labour.

often the shoulders will be raised. If the shoulders are raised, the scapula will also be raised, and so too will the tip of the inferior angle. An incorrect location of the spinous processes will result.

If the shoulders or arms are positioned forwards, the tip of the scapula will rotate around the chest wall. Again an incorrect location of the spinous processes will occur. Therefore, before locating the inferior angle of the scapula, position the shoulders into a position of ease. They must not be raised tensely or depressed unnaturally. The shoulder must not be protracted or retracted (not curved forwards or backwards). The arms should be positioned at the side of the body and not, for example, positioned forwards resting on a pillow. The distance between each pair of electrodes must be greater than the cross-sectional diameter of the electrodes.

Lower pair of electrodes. The lower pair of electrodes must be positioned on either side of the spine between S2 and S4. Palpate both sides of the lower back to find the top of the iliac crests of the pelvis. The fourth lumbar spinous process can be located by tracing an imaginary line from the top of the iliac crest to the midline. Using fingertips palpate slowly down over the fifth lumbar spinous process onto the sacral spines of S1, S2, S3 and S4. The electrodes must be positioned equally between S2 and S4. The sacral dimples are located over the posterior superior iliac spine which is at a level of S2. Once again the distance between the pair of electrodes should be greater than the cross-sectional diameter of the electrodes.

USING AN OBSTETRIC TENS UNIT

As previously highlighted, the various obstetric TENS units produced may offer slightly different facilities, so I would recommend referring to the step by step guides and/or videos which may be produced for each unit by the manufacturer. It should be remembered that each manufacturer's guidelines are for that unit only, and information provided should not be used generally for any TENS unit.

Ideally the TENS unit should provide sufficient intensity/amplitude to relieve labour pain. It should provide the facility to alter frequency (rate) according to individual preference, and also an ability to change from burst to continuous mode with an additional boost of amplitude. The frequency boost hand control should have a 'press/release' mechanism, not 'press/hold'. In addition it is desirable to have separate intensity controls for each pair of electrodes.

Introducing TENS to women

As this is a form of pain relief that can be applied and used at home it is extremely important that the woman and her partner understand exactly how to use the TENS unit effectively and safely. Time can be provided in antenatal preparation sessions. Ideally TENS talks and demonstrations should be available to provide advice and guidance as required. Information should be given in a sensitive way, within a relaxed atmosphere.

For some women the terminology 'electrical stimulation' conjures up thoughts of electric shock treatment. I have known women who expected the TENS unit to be plugged into the mains voltage! Rather than talking in terms of 'electric shocks' passing across the surface of the skin, the phrase 'packets of electrical energy' often conveys the message with empathy. In my experience this will allay the fears and anxieties of many individuals.

Women will be using the TENS unit in labour with the electrodes positioned on their backs, not on their forearms or between their fingers. Therefore, when introducing TENS to women, they should ideally be allowed to have the electrodes placed in the actual position in which they will be using the apparatus. Fingers and thumbs are very sensitive areas of the body and the sensation produced by the TENS when holding the electrodes may feel unpleasant and even painful.

If, during these sessions, partners are present then they can be shown the correct positioning for the electrodes. Permanent markers can be used to indicate the correct position for the electrodes on the skin. Women must be advised that TENS can help to modify the perception of pain in labour but will not eliminate pain sensation entirely. It can be safely used with other pain coping strategies such as relaxation, changing positions and breathing awareness. It should not be used by someone who is under hypnosis or is in a birthing pool. However it is safe to use before entering or after leaving a birthing pool. Aromatherapy essential oils may be used to fragrance the room at the same time as the TENS unit is being used. Care must, however, be taken not to allow any massage oils to come into contact with the electrodes if essential oils are being applied to the skin during a massage.

SUMMARY

For the physiotherapist who specialises in the field of obstetrics, TENS is a valuable therapy to utilise in appropriate circumstances. However, it must always be remembered that it is a form of pain relief, it does not treat the cause of pain. It is the objective of the physiotherapist to diagnose the cause of pain using assessment and examination. It is then possible to initiate treatment using a variety of therapies including specific exercise programmes, back care and posture correction, manipulation techniques, therapeutic massage, relaxation techniques and electrotherapy (ultrasound, pulsed electromagnetic energy, interferential laser therapy—note, however, that these are contraindicated in pregnancy). TENS may be used in conjunction with these modalities to provide analgesia only.

A midwife will advise women how to use TENS as part of her normal clinical practice as a method of pain relief in labour. It is important, however, for a midwife to be aware of the obstetric physiotherapist's role within the multidisciplinary team so that she can refer appropriately. Physiotherapists are qualified and competent to use TENS following the first trimester of pregnancy for many conditions.

In my experience TENS is a very valuable therapy to treat a variety of painful conditions experienced by women in both the antenatal and postnatal periods, as well as during labour. For example, I found it highly effective in treating, in consultation with medical colleagues, an antenatal client who was diagnosed as having fractured several ribs following a fall. She was 26 weeks pregnant and was experiencing severe chest pain. Myers et al (1977) have also reported highly effective results using TENS for treating traumatic injury, as in the case of fractured ribs.

I frequently find TENS invaluable in helping to alleviate the painful condition known as pubic symphisis diastasis. This condition can cause such pain that the client has great difficulty bearing weight and may even require hospitalisation. In other conditions, such as sacroiliac joint arthropathies and acute coccyx pain, TENS can provide valuable pain relief. I have also successfully treated a woman of 31 weeks gestation who had received severe burns some months earlier. A combination of the pressure garments used to treat her burns, the keloid scarring, inflamed and irritating skin and a very hot summer was making her pain intolerable. She found that TENS helped to modify her pain to a satisfactory level. I have also found TENS to be effective for treating the pain experienced by a client who was 27 weeks pregnant and suffered a fractured ilium following a fall.

In the postnatal period, TENS has a place for providing pain relief for differing conditions. TENS has provided valuable pain relief around the incision site for a number of women who have had a Caesarean birth. Hymes et al (1974) reported successful results in treating postoperative pain with TENS. When used postoperatively for pain relief, TENS does not produce the common side-effects associated with the use of narcotics, such as sedation, respiratory depression, and it has no undesirable effects on bowel motility. Several studies have shown TENS to reduce narcotic requirements postoperatively (Pike 1978, Rosenberg et al 1978, Solomon et al 1980, Ali et al 1981).

REFERENCES

Ali et al 1981 The effect of transcutaneous electrical nerve stimulation on post-operative pain and pulmonary function. Surgery 89: 507–512

Association of Chartered Physiotherapists in Obstetrics and Gynaecology 1992 The TENS Working Party 71: 22

Augustinsson P, Bohlin P, Bundsen P, Carlsson C, Forssman L, Sjoberg P, Tyreman N U 1977 Pain relief during labour by transcutaneous electrical nerve stimulation. Pain 4: 59–65

Browning A, Butt W, Lynch S, Shakespear R, Crawford J 1983 Maternal and cord plasma concentrations of beta lipotrophin, beta endorphin and gammalipotrophin at delivery: effect of analgesia. British Journal of Obstetrics and Gynaecology 99: 1152–1154

Bundsen P, Ericson K 1982 Pain relief in Labour by transcutaneous electrical nerve stimulation, safety aspects. Acta Obstet Gynecol Scandinavica 61: 1–5

Bundsen P, Peterson L, Selstam U 1981 Pain relief in labour by transcutaneous electrical nerve stimulation: a prospective matched study. Acta Obstet Gynecol Scandinavica 60: 459–468

Bundsen P, Ericson K, Peterson L, Thiringar C 1982 Pain relief in labour by transcutaneous electrical nerve stimulation: testing of a modified stimulation technique and evaluation of the neurological and biochemical condition of the newborn infant. Acta Obstet Gynecol Scandinavica 61: 129–136

Collins W, Randt C 1958 Evoked central nervous system activity relating to peripheral unmyelinated 'C' fibres in the cat. Journal of Neurophysiology 21: 345

Crawford J S 1984 Obstetric analgesia and anaesthesia, 2nd ed. No 1 in the series Current Reviews in Obstetrics and Gynaecology. Churchill Livingstone, Edinburgh.

Davies R J 1989 An evaluation of TENS pain relief in labour. Association of Chartered Physiotherapists in Obstetrics and Gynaecology 65: 2–7

Ericksson M, Schuller H, Sjolund B 1978 Hazard from transcutaneous nerve stimulators in patients with pacemakers. Lancet 1: 1319

Erkkola R, Pikkola P, Kanto J 1980 Transcutaneous nerve stimulation for pain relief during labour: a controlled study. Annales Cherurgiae et Gynaecologiae 69: 273–277

Fall M, Carlsson C, Erlandson B Electrical stimulation in interstitial cystitis. Journal of Urology 123: 192

Hagbarth K, Derr R 1954 Central influences on spinal afferent conduction. Journal of Neurophysiology 17: 295

Harrison R, Woods T, Shore M, Mathews G, Unwin A 1986 Pain relief in labour using transcutaneous electrical nerve stimulation: a tens/tens-placebo controlled study in two parity groups. British Journal of Obstetrics and Gynaecology 93: 139–146

Harrison R, Shore T, Mathews G, Gardiner J, Unwin A 1987 A comparative study of transcutaneous electrical nerve stimulation, Entonox, pethidine and promazine and lumbar epidural for pain relief in labour. Acta Obstet Gynaecol Scand 66: 9–14

Hymes A 1984 A review of the historical uses of electricity. In: Lampe G, Mannheimer J (eds) Clinical transcutaneous electrical nerve stimulation. FA Davis Company, Philadelphia

Hymes A C, Raab D E, Yonchiro E G, Nelson D G, Drintz A L 1974 Acute pain control by electrostimulation: a preliminary report. In: Bonica J J (ed) Advances in neurology 4. Ravensbury Press, New York, p 761–773

Janco M, Trontelj J 1980 TENS: a microneurographic and perceptual study. Pain 9: 219–230

Jones M 1980 Transcutaneous nerve stimulation in labour. Anaesthesia 35: 372–375

Kane K, Taub A 1975 A History of local electrical analgesia. Pain 1: 25–138

Kubista E, Kucera H, Riss P 1978 The effect of transcutaneous nerve stimulation on labour pain. Geburtshilfe Frauenheilkd 38: 1079

Lampe G, Mannheimer J 1984 Some limitations of TENS. In: Lampe G, Mannheimer J (eds) Clinical transcutaneous electrical nerve stimulation. FA Davis Company, Philadelphia

Long D 1974a Recent advances in the management of pain. Minn. Med 56: 705

Long D 1974b External electrical stimulation as treatment of chronic pain. Minn Med 57: 195

Melzack R, Wall P 1965 Pain mechanisms: a new theory. Science 150: 971

Melzack R, Wall P 1982 The challenge of pain. Penguin Books, London

Miller Jones C 1980 Transcutaneous nerve stimulation in Labour. Anaesthesia 35: 372–375

Myers R A, Woolf C J, Mitchell D 1977 Management of acute traumatic pain by peripheral transcutaneous electrical stimulation, South African Medical Journal 52: 309–312

Nathan P W 1976 The gate control theory of pain. A critical review. Brain 99: 123–158

Nesheim B I 1981 The use of transcutaneous nerve stimulation for pain relief during labour. Acta Obstet Gynecol Scand 60: 13–16

Neumark J, Pauser G, Scherzer W 1978 Pain relief in childbirth: an analysis of the analgesic effects of transcutaneous nerve stimulation, pethidine and placebos. Prakt Anaesth 13: 13

Pike P M 1978 Transcutaneous electrical stimulation: its use in the management of post-operative pain. Anaesthesia 33: 165–171

Poggio G F, Mountcastle V B 1960 A study of the functional contributions of the lemniscal and spinothalamic systems to somatic sensibility. Bulletin of Johns Hopkins Hospital: 106–266

Robson J E, Stewart P 1979 Transcutaneous nerve stimulation: a method of analgesia in labour. Anaesthesia 34: 357–364

Rockwell B, Byrd G M, Rockwell A D 1875 A practical treatise on the medical and surgical uses of electricity in Wood W, New York. 1875 Museum of Electricity in Life at Medtronic, Minneapolis

Rosenberg 1978 Transcutaneous electrical nerve stimulation for the relief of post-operative pain. Pain 5: 129–135

Salar G, Job I, Mingrino S, Bosio A, Trabucchi M 1981 Effects of transcutaneous electrotherapy on C S F beta endorphin content in patients without pain problems. Pain 10: 169–172

Shealy C N 1966 The physiological substrate of pain. Headache 6: 101

Shealy C N 1973 Transcutaneous electroanalgesia. Surgical Forum 23: 419

Shealy C N 1974 Six years' experience with electrical stimulation for the control of pain. Advanced Neurology 4: 775

Shealy C N, Maurer D 1974 Transcutaneous nerve stimulation for the control of pain. Surgical Neurology 2: 45–47

Sjolund B, Terenuis L, Eriksson M 1977 Increased cerebrospinal fluid levels of endorphins after electroacupuncture. Acta Physiologica Scandinavica 100: 382–384

Solomon 1980 Reduction of post-operative pain and narcotic use by transcutaneous electrical nerve stimulation. Surgery 87: 142–146

Tawfik O, Badraoui M H H, El Ridi F S 1982 The value of transcutaneous nerve stimulation during labour in Egyptian mothers. Schmertz: 98–105

Thompson J W 1988 Pharmacology of transcutaneous electrical nerve stimulation. Intractable Pain Society 7 (1): 33–40

Thorsteinsson G, Stonnington H H, Stillwell G K 1977 Transcutaneous electrical stimulation. A double blind trial of its efficacy of pain. Arch Phys. Med. Rehab 58: 8–13

UKCC 1991 Registrar's letter 8/1991 14/5/91. UKCC, London

UKCC 1994 The midwife's code of practice. UKCC, London

Wall P D 1967 The laminar organization of the dorsal horn and effects of descending impulses. Journal of Physiology 188: 403

Woolf C J 1994 Transcutaneous and implanted nerve stimulation. In: Wall P, Melzack R (eds) Textbook of pain. Churchill Livingstone, Edinburgh, p 679–690

FURTHER INFORMATION

Obstetric TENS unit manufacturers

1. Neen Health Care
   Old Pharmacy Yard
   Church Street
   Dereham
   Norfolk
   NR19 1DJ
   England
   Tel: 01362 698966

This company has been producing the 'Microtens' Obstetric Unit. Recently they have produced a new unit to be used in labour and it is called the 'Lifetime Microtens'. The company has a rental-hire scheme and offers a package for health professionals.

2. Promedics Limited
   Clarendon Road
   Blackburn
   Lancashire
   BB1 9TA
   England
   Tel: 01254 57700

This company produces the 'SPECTRUM' obstetric TENS unit and offers a rental-hire scheme. They include an instructional video. The company offers a package for professionals.

3. Spembly Medical
   Newbury Road
   Andover
   Hampshire
   SP10 4DR
   England
   Tel: 01264 365 741
   Care-line freephone: 0800 515413

This company produces the 'Pulsar' Obstetric TENS unit. They offer a rental-hire scheme and also a package for health professionals. They have also produced an instructional video.

4. Raymar
   Unit One, Fairview Estate
   Henley on Thames
   Oxon
   RG9 1HE
   Tel: 01491 578446
   Fax: 01491 410233

This company produces 'BabiTens' obstetric TENS unit. The company offers rental package schemes.

11

Drugs in labour

Ruth Bevis

LEARNING OUTCOMES

At the end of this chapter the reader will have

- **an increased awareness of the responsibilities of the midwife in relation to the administration of drugs in labour**

- **an increased awareness of the pharmacological methods of pain relief used at various stages of labour**

- **an increased understanding of the use of narcotic agents and the implications of misuse to both the mother and fetus/infant**

- **identified the routes of administration of drugs in labour, including patient controlled analgesia (PCA)**

- **identified analgesic and anaesthetic agents used for pain relief in labour**

- **considered relief of pain after Caesarean section, and in the immediate postnatal period.**

THE MIDWIFE IN THE UK AND THE ADMINISTRATION OF DRUGS

The midwife has a unique role in her care of women in labour. She has to ensure that both mother and fetus receive optimal care, planned to meet their specific needs, and giving full consideration to the wishes of the woman and her partner. Both women and midwives are protected by legislation, from which arise the *Midwives' Rules* and *Professional Code of Practice*, drawn up by the

United Kingdom Central Council for Nursing, Midwifery and Health Visiting (UKCC). The midwife must be fully conversant with each of these and must keep abreast of new developments and current law. She must also be clear about her own remit for giving drugs within local standing orders agreed by the obstetric team and must clearly understand the responsibility this carries. Every midwife must be aware of and must adhere to legislation relating to prescribing, storage, handling and checking of all types of drugs, including controlled drugs (CDs). In addition, she must follow local protocols in regard to these.

The law

The Acts of Parliament relating to the midwife's practice include:

- Medicines Act 1968
- Misuse of Drugs Act 1971
- Misuse of Drugs Regulations 1985
- Misuse of Drugs Act (1971)–Modification Order 1985
- Medicines (Prescriptions Only) Order 1983

The UKCC

Arising from these various statutes are national standards governing practice. These include:

- *Midwives' Rules* and *A Midwife's Code of Practice* (UKCC 1993, 1994)
- *Standards for the Administration of Medicines* (UKCC 1992).

The *Midwives' Rules* state that: 'A practising midwife shall not on her own responsibility administer any medicine, including analgesics, unless in the course of her training, whether before or after registration as a midwife, she has been thoroughly instructed in its use and is familiar with its dosage and methods of administration or application.'

If any midwife feels she is not adequately trained in any such area of practice, it is her responsibility to acquire suitable training.

Standing orders and protocols

These are agreed between senior midwives, obstetricians, anaesthetists, paediatricians and pharmacy staff, and take into account the local situation—the availability of obstetric and anaesthetic staff, the population and their perceived needs, and the preferences and beliefs of the midwifery and medical staff involved. Such standing orders will normally state the drugs which may be given by a midwife, without a prescription, to women at any stage of pregnancy, during labour or in the puerperium. They will state the circumstances, the route, dosage, frequency of administration and the maximum number of doses which may be given. Midwives working in other countries will be subject to similar legislation and guidelines.

Many women require analgesic and other drugs in labour. The main problem with medication for the pregnant woman is the unique situation of two subjects—mother and fetus. Almost any substance ingested by the woman will cross the placental barrier, some to a greater and others to a lesser extent. The concern is clearly that the fetus should not be harmed in the short or the long term by the treatment given to the mother. Drugs given in labour and entering the maternal circulation will cross the placental barrier to and from the fetus, following the concentration gradient. This means that when the fetal circulation contains a higher concentration of a drug than the maternal circulation, the drug will start to diffuse back across into the maternal circulation and vice versa. Some drugs will be wholly or partly metabolised by the fetal liver or kidneys, while others may cross the blood–brain barrier and exert some pharmacological effect on the fetus or neonate.

EARLY LABOUR

The main requirements of the woman in early labour are relief of pain and alleviation of anxiety. She may also need sleep, but meeting the first two needs may enable her to do this. In the UK it is no longer usual to give sedatives, such as chloral derivatives, which were commonly used until the

1980s, often with a mild analgesic such as para-cetamol. Paracetamol may still be given in the very early stages, before labour becomes established. However, reassurance and supportive companionship will go a long way towards reducing anxiety. Pleasant surroundings and a calm, friendly midwife who gives the woman the opportunity to ask questions and spends time answering them appropriately will help still further. The midwife may not always feel relaxed herself, particularly if she is very busy, but it is part of the professionalism required of her that she should not allow this to affect her standard of care.

NARCOTIC DRUGS

A narcotic drug is a strong analgesic with some sedative properties, and these include the opioids. 'Opioid' is a broader term than the older 'opiate', which refers solely to morphine-like drugs having a similar chemical structure to morphine. There are now a number of peptides and synthetic analogues which resemble morphine in action but not in structure (Herz 1993). The term opioid refers to all these substances.

The body produces its own endogenous opioids (endorphins and enkephalins) and this production is increased in situations of pain or stress, such as labour or sustained strenuous exercise. There are opioid receptors throughout the central nervous system, in particular in the brain and throughout the length of the spinal cord. Three types of specific opioid receptor are described, plus a fourth which is not purely an opioid receptor. Different opioids bind to the various receptors with differing degrees of affinity, giving rise to the various opioid effects, wanted and unwanted. These include analgesia, sedation, euphoria, respiratory depression, reduction in gastrointestinal motility, dysphoria (hallucinations and unpleasant dreams and sensations) and physical dependence, all in varying degrees. The analgesia produced will vary in different circumstances, such as acute and chronic pain. Nociception is defined as the perception of noxious stimuli, which is not necessarily pain. Opioids will have an effect on nociception, and will often reduce the distress associated with pain, although the subject will not always describe a significant reduction in the actual pain sensation (Rang et al 1995).

Agonist and antagonist effects

An agonist is a drug which combines with an opioid receptor and gives rise to a biological opioid effect including analgesia. The best known examples of opioid agonist analgesic agents are morphine and pethidine. An antagonist binds to the receptor 'in competition' with the opioid agonist and so blocks its effect. This is important because it enables unwanted effects to be reversed. The commonly used example in obstetrics is naloxone, given to prevent or reverse respiratory depression in either the mother or the neonate. The baby may be given naloxone at delivery, or it may be given to the mother prior to delivery, the former being more specific and effective. Another unwanted effect is itching after the administration of epidural or spinal opioids. Naloxone will reverse this unpleasant side-effect, but it will also reverse the effect of the analgesia. If given alone, in the absence of another opioid, it will have no obvious effect.

Some drugs exhibit both agonist and antagonist effects. An example of one which has been used in obstetrics is pentazocine, which may cause dysphoria and has never gained wide popularity. Its analgesic effect has not been shown to be superior to that of pethidine.

Opioids in labour

Pethidine. A number of opioid drugs have been studied for their efficacy in labour, but the drug which has been used consistently since 1940 is pethidine (meperidine, Pamergan). Although it is regarded with scepticism by some because of its unwanted effects on the neonate, it remains a useful drug. Like any other drug its effects will be slightly different for different subjects. It may cause some women to be more sleepy and detached from reality than others. Some women may like this effect, and find they can relax and doze between contractions. Others, who wish to be fully alert and in control throughout labour, are not likely to find pethidine their ideal analgesic. However, judicious use of a smaller dose, even in these women, may just relieve the acuteness of their pain so that they may cope well. Some women will complain of nausea, and may vomit after pethidine.

Pethidine will begin to give some analgesia as soon as 10 minutes after intramuscular injection; it will reach maximum effect after 1 hour and then gradually decline. A second dose given during labour will therefore boost a background analgesia remaining from the first dose, giving some cumulative effect.

Its use is governed by standing orders in most obstetric units in the UK, and midwives may usually give between 50 and 150 mg by intramuscular injection. The higher dose is normally allowed once only, and after this only 100 mg is permitted. There will also be a limit on the total dose given, and on the frequency of use. These safeguards are in place for the protection of midwives as well as mothers. It may mean that 100 mg is given to all women, regardless of their size, when a large woman will clearly need 150 mg, and a small, slim woman may only need 75 mg, and an experienced midwife will interpret the standing orders thoughtfully. Any analgesic requirements which are outside of the standing orders should be discussed with the doctor, who may prescribe or recommend some other course of action.

There is a general belief that pethidine should not be given within 2–4 hours of delivery because of an increased risk of neonatal respiratory depression. Reynolds (1990b) refutes this and states that it is barbaric to withhold analgesia at this stage if it is required. Morrison et al (1973) showed that the neonatal effects are greater if pethidine is given several hours before delivery and negligible if given 1 hour beforehand. Kuhnert et al (1985) replicated this finding while looking at the effects of low doses of pethidine. Most standing orders would probably be found to reflect this general belief rather than the quoted research findings.

The midwife is of course free to request epidural analgesia for her client where appropriate, but the anaesthetist may not wish to give epidural opioids after a woman has been given systemic opioids, because of the risk of respiratory depression and possible cumulative or delayed effects.

Pethidine may be used in conjunction with other drugs, such as metoclopramide and promethazine or promazine (see p. 153). Its use continues to be debated, and there is general agreement that the search for the ideal analgesic for labour should continue (Reynolds 1990b, Thomson et al 1994).

Morphine. Morphine was the first opioid drug widely used for labour, apart from opium itself. It gives good analgesia, plus sedation and euphoria. It has a longer duration of action than pethidine, and causes more respiratory depression in the baby. It is little used for systemic analgesia in labour today.

Diamorphine. This gives good analgesia, sedation and euphoria, but fears of addiction and its effect on the baby make it an unsuitable drug for general obstetric use in the opinion of the majority of medical staff. However the National Birthday Trust Fund (NBT) survey found similar percentages of women using diamorphine and meptazinol (3.6% and 3.3%, respectively, as reported in the midwives' questionnaires). It is perhaps surprising that diamorphine is so widely used in view of its association with drug addiction (Steer 1990). The study does not give a clear indication as to how many units use it as the regular opioid for labour, or whether a large number of units used it occasionally.

Meptazinol. Meptazinol (Meptid) is given by intramuscular injection in doses of 100 or 150 mg. It has the advantage of causing fewer side-effects than other opioid drugs. It does not cause significant respiratory depression, or euphoria or dysphoria. It does cause nausea and vomiting, and has some atropine-like effects. Its analgesic effect is very similar to that of pethidine (Sheikh & Tunstall 1986, Osler 1987). Its effect on the baby is reported to be minimal, since it is better metabolised by the neonate (Morgan 1982). The findings of the National Birthday Trust Fund survey (Chamberlain et al 1993) seem to indicate that this may not be entirely true; the data, however, are obtained from a retrospective postal survey, and look only at Apgar scores.

Pentazocine. Pentazocine (Fortral) was welcomed as the ideal obstetric analgesic drug some years ago, but proved disappointing. Its analgesic efficacy is similar to that of pethidine, with a dosage of 40 mg equating to 100 mg of pethidine, and the usual maximum dose being 60 mg. The incidence of nausea and vomiting is less than with pethidine, but dysphoria and sweating are common complaints.

General indications for the use of opioids by the midwife

The midwife must be aware of local standing orders and protocols, and understand the details of the drug administration that is within her remit. The woman should be in established labour.

Opioids are generally believed to be best avoided within 4 hours of the anticipated time of delivery, and certainly within 2 hours. Some studies appear to refute this (see discussion on p. 152). Many standing orders are still based on this belief, and may only allow pethidine to be given in the late first stage at the discretion of a senior midwife, since the effects on the baby are largely reversible by giving naloxone (see p. 151).

Every midwife must ensure that the woman gives informed consent to receiving an opioid drug. Informed consent is a difficult issue once a woman is distressed, in pain and tired, since she may not be capable of listening, understanding information and asking questions. It may be argued that the only valid informed consent is obtained at the end of pregnancy, but a woman may find the labour experience so far from her expectations that she may jettison her birth plan completely (Rickford & Reynolds 1987). In addition, the labouring woman's partner may have promised her beforehand that he/she will support her in her wishes, and the midwife may therefore have to negotiate a route acceptable to all.

Other routes for the administration of opioids

While the midwife in the UK will only be giving opioids by the intramuscular route on her own responsibility, such drugs are also used in the epidural space, the subarachnoid space (see Chapter 12), and intravenously.

Patient controlled analgesia (PCA). Some centres may give intravenous opioids on a carefully regulated self-administration basis. This involves a dilute solution of opioid in normal saline which is available to the woman in a controlled dose at preset intervals. Women generally like the control this gives them, but American studies have shown that this results in higher total doses and more fetal effects (Rayburn et al 1989) compared with a carefully controlled nurse-administered procedure, and McIntosh & Rayburn (1991) found it generally inadequate for labour, but satisfactory for postoperative pain.

Drugs used with opioids

Drug combinations in labour are given with the main aims of:

- potentiating the analgesic effects of opioids so that a lower total dose is needed
- reducing nausea and vomiting
- reducing gastric contents by improving gastric emptying
- reducing gastric acid production
- reducing the acidity of existing gastric contents.

The drugs used to achieve these effects are the phenothiazine derivatives, promethazine and promazine. These are said to potentiate the analgesic effect and reduce nausea and vomiting. Combined with an opioid they may make the woman more drowsy than the opioid alone. Vella et al (1985) compared promethazine and metoclopramide, and found that promethazine tended to antagonise the analgesic effect, while increasing drowsiness.

Metoclopramide is an anti-emetic drug, which increases gastric motility without stimulating gastric acid production. It is an effective adjunct to pethidine in reducing nausea and vomiting.

Certain drugs known as H_2 receptor antagonists are commonly used in labour, for example ranitidine and cimetidine. They inhibit the production of gastric acid and so raise gastric pH, although they do not neutralise existing gastric acid. They may be given to any woman with moderate or high risk factors in labour. The concern is that if the woman needs a general anaesthetic for Caesarean section, regurgitation of acid stomach contents during induction of anaesthesia may cause acid aspiration into the lungs, leading to Mendelson's syndrome, which is a significant cause of maternal morbidity and death (Bevis 1984, Report on the confidential enquiry into maternal morbidity and mortality 1985–1987). Some anaesthetists believe that ranitidine should always be given with pethidine because they are concerned that pethidine causes significant delay in gastric emptying (Reynolds 1993). Famotidine is a new drug in this class, which is very effective and has the added advantage of reducing gastric contents. At the time of writing it is not in use in obstetrics, but is viewed with interest by obstetric anaesthetists.

Antacids are now used less frequently and are given to neutralise acid stomach contents, for the same reasons. They may be given to all women in labour, or used selectively. The antacid first used routinely was mist magnesium trisilicate, but it was found that its particulate composition led to problems if aspiration of stomach contents occurred. The antacid in most common use at the present time is sodium citrate although its action is fairly short-lived (Reynolds 1990a, Browne & Powell 1993).

DRUGS AND THE FETUS AND NEONATE

Most drugs given to the pregnant woman will cross the placental barrier to some extent—an important exception is heparin. The effects on the fetus may be considered under the headings of immediate, short-term and long-term. Immediate effects may be seen in the example of lignocaine used in paracervical block, where an immediate fetal bradycardia may occur. Short-term effects include the respiratory depression of the neonate when the mother has been given opioids in labour, and the more subtle neurobehavioural effects which last over the first days and weeks of the baby's life.

Long-term effects include teratogenicity from some drugs in pregnancy, two classic examples being thalidomide, causing limb defects, and alcohol causing fetal alcohol syndrome (FAS). Streptomycin and gentamicin may affect the auditory nerve, leading to deafness, and tetracyclines are known to stain the child's teeth brown or yellow.

A study that may cause concern for many people has suggested that women given relatively large amounts of opioid and barbiturate drugs in labour between 1945 and 1966 had a higher incidence of children who became drug addicts (Jacobsen et al 1990). The hypothesis is that the opioids given in labour had an 'imprinting' effect which predisposed those children to become addicted in later life. It is important to recognise that there was no regional anaesthesia in the 1940s–1960s, often very little emotional support in labour in the earlier part of that period, and women were given relatively large quantities of narcotic drugs to sedate them and keep them quiet, often resulting in total amnesia of the labour.

In a long labour, where Caesarean section was very much a last resort, much higher total doses would be given than would be considered appropriate by today's standards. The paper studied babies born in Stockholm, but the pattern of care was probably similar to that in the UK at the time. Happily, there are alternatives in the 1990s, and many changes in attitude, so that every woman should be able to have care and analgesia which is satisfactory to her. This paper gives good reason for caution in drug administration at any stage of pregnancy. National and international standards of drug testing are very stringent, and all drugs licensed in the UK will have undergone rigorous trials.

Neurobehavioural scores

Brazelton (1973) studied the subtle effects of opioids on the baby in the first few days of life during the early 1970s. He recognised that a rough assessment of the baby's condition at birth was an inadequate measure. He looked at factors such as response to light and sound, primitive reflexes such as the Moro reflex, cuddliness and consolability. He also measured frequency of sucking, peak pressure of sucking during feeding, and total milk consumption. He found lower scores in babies of mothers who had received systemic opioids.

Kuhnert et al (1985) found that even low doses of pethidine gave significantly lower neuro-behavioural scores in the babies than in babies of mothers who had received no medication. The researchers looked at cuddliness, consolability, quieting and hand-to-mouth activity. These factors have clear implications for the establishment of breast feeding, early social interaction, and the mother's feelings about her baby and her ability to care for him. It has been suggested that pethidine also interferes with the baby's ability to migrate towards the breast shortly after delivery (Rajan 1994).

The use of naloxone

Naloxone has already been discussed as a useful opioid antagonist which may be given to the baby at delivery to reverse respiratory depression following administration of pethidine to the mother during labour. It is important that the midwife is aware that naloxone has a short half-life, so that it may become ineffective before the opioid metabolite has been excreted by the baby, who may then start to exhibit opioid effects again. A short half-life of naloxone also occurs in the mother, so if she has been given the drug the opioid effects may be resumed after a period of time. The half-life of a drug is the time taken for the plasma concentration to decrease by half.

INHALATION ANALGESIA

Midwives in the UK may assist mothers in the use of Entonox provided they have been trained to do so. They must be conversant with the mode of action of Entonox and its administration, and must have been suitably trained and supervised in the use of the equipment. The equipment in turn must be one of the models approved by the UKCC for use by the midwife without medical supervision. It must be properly maintained and serviced at the prescribed intervals. There are four models currently approved for use by midwives:

- the BOC Entonox equipment (see Fig. 11.1)
- the PneuPac apparatus
- the SOS Nitronox–midwifery model
- the Peacemaker.

Entonox is a mixture of nitrous oxide and oxygen in equal parts. Nitrous oxide is an anaesthetic gas when mixed with a lower proportion of oxygen, such as in the ratio 70:30, and is commonly used as the maintenance agent in general anaesthesia. It is colourless and odourless.

In the delivery suite Entonox is usually available to each room in a piped supply. In this case the supply is supervised at the central bank by maintenance staff. There is a theoretical risk to staff from excessive exposure to nitrous oxide, and so exhaled Entonox may be removed from the delivery room via scavenging equipment.

A smaller type of cylinder may be used on a movable stand. The Entonox apparatus is not interchangeable with any other medical gas cylinder. Cylinders and equipment match up with a different pattern of pins and holes for each gas—the BOC pin index system. Every medical gas is supplied in a cylinder of a specific colour. An Entonox cylinder is always blue, with a blue and white quartered 'shoulder'.

If the midwife is using Entonox equipment in a domiciliary setting she needs to be familiar with handling and care of gas cylinders. They should be stored in clean, dry conditions, preferably inside and not subjected to extremes of heat or cold. No smoking or naked flames should be permitted within the vicinity of cylinders. Entonox is non-flammable but does support combustion. It is highly dangerous if in contact with oils, greases, tarry substances and many plastics, due to the risk of spontaneous combustion with high pressure gases (BOC gases). The nitrous oxide and oxygen gas mixture begins to separate if the cylinders have been subjected to temperatures below −7°C, because of what is known as the 'Poynting' effect. At that temperature nitrous oxide reverts to a liquid state and separates out from oxygen which is a gas. The cylinder must subsequently be stored horizontally for 24 hours at a temperature above 10°C. A mixture is then obtained by agitating the cylinder.

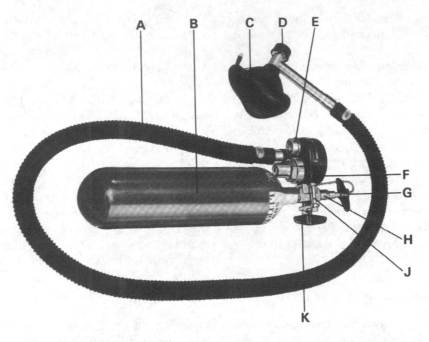

Figure 11.1 BOC Entonox analgesic apparatus (as used in the home). A, corrugated rubber tubing; B, 500 litre cylinder; C, face mask; D, expiratory valve; E, cylinder pressure gauge; F, demand regulator; G, cylinder valve key; H, pin index valve; J, cylinder yoke; K, cylinder yoke key. (Reproduced with the kind permission of Bennet & Brown 1993.)

Entonox has its effect very quickly, within approximately 20 seconds, reaching a maximum level at about 45–60 seconds. It is completely excreted from the body in a very short time when the woman stops using it, and is therefore thought not to have any measurable effect on the fetus. It should be used on a self-administration basis, so that if the woman becomes too sleepy she will drop the mask or mouth-piece and will not be over-sedated.

The woman has to extract the gas from the apparatus by her inspiratory effort; the gas does not flow out freely. She should be instructed to fit the mask firmly over her face, around her nose and mouth, and to inhale steadily as soon as she feels the start of a contraction. She should continue until the peak of the contraction has passed. In this way she will obtain maximum benefit.

Women who do not find Entonox a satisfactory method of analgesia are often afraid to use it to the full potential, and need clear instruction and encouragement. Some women will feel claustrophobic using the mask, and may complain about the smell of the black rubber tubing. They may prefer to use a small plastic mouthpiece which is also available. The principle is the same: the woman is instructed to close her lips firmly around the mouthpiece and breathe in the same way. There is an expiratory valve on the Entonox apparatus, so she does not need to remove the mask or mouthpiece during a contraction to exhale. She should be encouraged not to hyperventilate. Signs of this include dizziness and tingling of the hands and face.

Although some women dislike Entonox, and are not satisfied by the level of pain relief it gives, it still has a place in obstetric analgesia, particularly where the woman just needs a little help at the end of the first stage of labour. It may be used with opioids or as a simple adjunct to any other form of analgesia if this alone becomes inadequate.

Other inhalation analgesics used by UK midwives in the past, are trichloroethylene (Trilene) and methoxyflurane (Penthrane) but these are no longer approved by the UKCC (Bevis 1984). A combination of Entonox and isoflurane, a volatile anaesthetic agent, has been tried on a small sample of women and found to be effective, but this would be for administration under medical supervision (Wee et al 1993).

LOCAL ANAESTHETICS

Local infiltration

The local anaesthetic agent most commonly used by midwives is lignocaine. Its onset of action is fairly rapid, with a short duration of action, and it is used to infiltrate the perineum prior to performing an episiotomy or suturing. The mode of action of local anaesthetic agents is described in Chapter 12. The midwife is normally permitted to give a total dose of 50 mg either as 5 ml of 1% lignocaine or 10 ml of 0.5% solution.

Midwives need to be aware that there is a risk of toxicity if 200 mg is given, as an excessive amount will be absorbed systemically. Inadvertent intravenous injection can cause symptoms similar to those of toxicity which may include numbness of the tongue and around the mouth, a feeling of light-headedness, dizziness and tinnitus. Drowsiness and twitching may then occur and eventually lead to generalised convulsions, which may be rapidly fatal. The premonitory signs may be absent or occur so quickly that the first warning sign is drowsiness.

The principles in infiltration of the perineum are to await good analgesia from the infiltration before performing the procedure (episiotomy or suturing) and to avoid inadvertent intravenous injection.

Topical application

A recent study (Collins et al 1994) examined the efficacy of 2% lignocaine gel applied to the perineum during the second stage in reducing post-delivery perineal pain. It appeared to have a significant effect and merits further study. It would provide non-invasive analgesia with no side-effects other than possibly a local sensitivity reaction in some women, and could be provided by midwives.

Pudendal block

Pudendal block is not widely used since rapid analgesia for instrumental delivery may be provided with a spinal block. It may be useful in certain situations. The obstetrician injects lignocaine transvaginally through a long, guarded needle to anaesthetise both branches of the pudendal nerve. This lies adjacent to the ischial spines, and just beyond the sacrospinous ligament. The perineum is also infiltrated with local anaesthetic, and this should give adequate if not ideal analgesia in skilled hands, for a low forceps or Ventouse delivery.

Paracervical block

This type of block is not often used and was never widely used in the UK, though it was popular in the USA. It blocks the pain of cervical dilatation, though not of contractions or perineal stretching. The aim is to block the paracervical plexus. The local anaesthetic is given transvaginally through a long, guarded needle, injecting the solution into the lateral fornices. There is a significant risk of intravenous injection or simply systemic absorption due to vascularity, leading to fetal bradycardia. Lignocaine or bupivacaine may be used.

The effect is not long-lived if lignocaine is used, and so the process may have to be repeated; it is invasive and disruptive, and therefore not generally acceptable. A recent paper concluded that the technique can be useful, but should be avoided in any situation where the fetus is already at risk, such as intrauterine growth retardation or any signs of fetal distress (Ranta et al 1995).

PAIN RELIEF AFTER CAESAREAN SECTION

Immediate care

Relief of pain in the immediate postpartum period is an aspect of midwifery practice which is difficult to separate from relief of pain in labour, as one so frequently impinges on the other. Attention is therefore drawn to this aspect of pain management, although it is not intended that this will be dealt with in any detail in this text. The care of women who have undergone Caesarean section, for example, will often be initiated whilst still in the labour ward. Continuity of care is therefore a factor midwives should consider, particularly as the woman is transferred to the postnatal ward for ongoing care. In addition, postnatal pain has already been identified as an area for extra consideration and evaluation in midwifery practice and therefore cannot be overstated (see p. 15).

Epidural top-up

Good analgesia after Caesarean section is essential to enable the woman to become mobile quickly in order to minimise postoperative complications. It will also enable her to care for the baby and enjoy the early days of their relationship. If an epidural was used during labour or Caesarean section she may have received a top-up of analgesia. An opioid top-up gives good analgesia (Leicht et al 1986) but there is a risk of respiratory depression, and her condition must be closely monitored, with at least hourly recording of respirations, and noting of any undue sleepiness (MacLeod 1993, Woods 1993). The latter is difficult to evaluate, since many women will feel tired after Caesarean section, especially if preceded by many hours in labour. The woman should be cared for in a recovery area if levels of care in the postnatal ward are in doubt. If adequate care is not available then opioid top-ups are not a safe option (MacLeod 1993). If a local anaesthetic top-up was given she will have impaired motor function and this must be properly assessed before she is mobilised. Full assessment of motor block includes testing for cold sensation, pin-prick and straight leg raising. The ideal top-up may be a combination so that side-effects from both types of drug are minimal, since a lower dose of both will be required.

Patient-controlled epidural anaesthesia (PCEA)

Patient-controlled epidural analgesia (PCEA) may be used for the immediate post-operative period, but the overriding consideration is the late onset or cumulative effect of respiratory depression (Davies et al 1980). Doses would be low and dilute, and women are reported to find this method very satisfactory (Gordon et al 1994).

Systemic analgesia

If there is no epidural catheter *in situ*, systemic analgesia will be prescribed. This should be given promptly, ideally anticipating the return of pain so as to minimise distress. If the prescribed dose is inadequate the midwife should seek medical advice.

Patient-controlled analgesia (PCA) may be used, with a low-dose, dilute solution given intravenously on demand.

When intramuscular (strong) analgesia is not required, some form of moderate analgesic will be prescribed. This may be oral or rectal. Analgesic suppositories such as diclofenac may be very useful in minimising gastrointestinal side-effects or where there is nausea or vomiting. Some women may dislike the route of administration, and their preference should be respected.

Comfort measures

Most women will feel much better in the immediate postoperative period once they have had the epidural catheter, urinary catheter and intravenous infusion removed. Organising help for the woman to wash, clean her teeth, brush her hair and put on her own clothes is an essential component of the midwifery role.

Apart from the surgical pain the woman is likely to have some discomfort from abdominal distension and 'wind'. A homely remedy such as hot peppermint water may be helpful alongside the prescribed analgesic. The gut is packed away from the uterus during surgery and a paralytic ileus is a possible complication. The woman must be observed for signs of increasing abdominal distension, pain and persistently absent bowel sounds, and appropriate action taken.

The use of caring skills and comfort measures such as helping the woman get into a comfortable position, particularly when feeding the baby, whether breast or bottle fed, will help to minimise the need for further analgesia. She may like to have her own pillows in order to achieve maximum comfort.

Care of bladder and bowels is an important element in postoperative comfort, particularly as opioid drugs may cause urinary retention (Woods 1993). The midwife should try to ensure that the woman gets adequate rest, since pain and discomfort will feel worse if she cannot get quality sleep.

PAIN IN THE POSTNATAL PERIOD

The midwife should ensure that women receive appropriate analgesic measures during the immediate postnatal period. She should use her midwifery skills to ensure that all pain and discomfort are alleviated as far as possible. This does not just involve regular dispensing of paracetamol.

Some of the causes of postnatal pain include 'after pains', or painful breasts as experienced at the time of initiation of lactation, and potentially sore nipples. It is important that adequate analgesia is provided, however every midwife should be aware of current practice relating to advising and assisting the breastfeeding mother. Advice relating to correct positioning of the baby, effective fixing and feeding regimes should be based on sound research-based practice. It is important for every midwife to be aware that sedation and analgesics given during labour may compromise the establishment of successful breastfeeding.

The postnatal period is a time when many of the complementary remedies may be helpful. Perineal pain may be treated with remedies such as a 'sitz' bath with marigold tincture as obtained from a herbalist, or sitting in a warm bath to which a small amount of witch hazel has been added. Many of the aromatherapy oils, such as lavender, are believed to be beneficial at this time; it will be helpful to be in contact with a local aromatherapist. Many health care professionals, including midwives, are becoming qualified in complementary techniques and may therefore be readily available in some areas for advice (see p. 111–112 for contact numbers). Severe bruising and oedema may require the physiotherapist's help with ultrasound treatment.

Haemorrhoids are another common cause of pain and discomfort in the postnatal period. Haemorrhoids may be very swollen and painful after a long second stage or instrumental delivery, and may require some topical treatment. The woman will also be fearful of the first bowel movement, and the midwife may need to offer suitable measures to ensure that the stool is soft. A bulking agent such as Fybogel may be sufficient; if it is not, a stool softening agent should be given. Fybogel is useful in preventing the pain of constipation in any newly delivered woman.

Urinary retention or difficulty with micturition may occur after operative delivery or, in particular, after an epidural using opioids, although any newly delivered woman may find some disturbance of bladder function. Immediate attention to this problem will alleviate the pain of urinary retention, and help prevent subsequent urinary tract infection.

THE NATIONAL BIRTHDAY TRUST FUND SURVEY

The National Birthday Trust Fund was set up in 1928, to look at maternity care across the country. Queen Mary herself viewed 'with grave concern the continued high rate of maternal mortality', which she saw as a 'reproach on our national life', and gave her full support to the NBT Fund. Much useful information has been gathered since 1928 giving indications of current trends across the UK.

Interestingly, the original aims of the Trust were:

- to make childbirth safer for mother and baby
- to promote the wider use of pain relief in labour
- to provide funds for the salaries of anaesthetists to cover maternity hospitals and for equipment for the greater improvement of pain relief.

The National Birthday Trust Fund has had very significant input, both in terms of persuading the establishment and in terms of funding, in most of the main developments in analgesia in midwifery practice.

During 1 week in June 1990, the NBT undertook a nation-wide survey on pain relief in labour. The study looked at the types of unit, staffing levels, the analgesic methods available, and those used. The study was a descriptive, prospective survey, using postal questionnaires. The initial questionnaire, branch 1, was sent to a senior midwife in every maternity unit in the country, asking for a profile of the unit. A total of 89% of units completed the entire survey. Branch 2A and branch 2B questionnaires were sent to midwives, and to all the women (and their partners) who delivered during the selected week. The midwife caring for each woman at the time of delivery was asked to complete the branch 2A questionnaire. The branch 3 questionnaire was sent to 10% of responding women 6 weeks after delivery, seeking their retrospective feelings about the labour.

The report on the survey gives interesting background information on the undertaking of such a large-scale study, describing some of the pitfalls and problems encountered. The research methodology is discussed. Findings are discussed, and data are presented in graphic form, for the most part easy to interpret quickly (Chamberlain et al 1993). Important information is extrapolated on the effect of different analgesic methods on the baby, and obstetric anaesthesia. An interesting dichotomy emerges between the midwife's perception of pain relief and that of the mother. Women under-reported the use of the less usual drugs such as meptazinol, presumably because they did not know what drug they had received. Midwives under-reported the use of relaxation techniques as an analgesic method compared with what was reported by the women. Does this indicate that they did not notice what the mother was doing, or that they undervalued it?

The recommendations of the report are very relevant to the politics and practicalities of maternity care. They include better education and information of women to prepare them for the pain of labour in a realistic way, audit of women's satisfaction with pain relief in every maternity unit, and looking at ways of reducing the side-effects of pethidine, especially in relation to breastfeeding.

SUMMARY

There is a suggestion that pain relief in labour is so fraught with danger that it should be avoided if at all possible (Wagner 1993). No compassionate midwife is going to sit back and watch women suffer unnecessarily, but she does have to weigh up the benefits and risks to each of her clients—mother and baby—every time she recommends or administers any form of analgesia (Haire 1993, Priest & Rosser 1991).

The midwife is required to keep abreast of current developments and research findings, and where these are not reflected in practice she should press for change, as well as undertaking and encouraging further research in this area. She must show compassion and empathy and develop her professional skills, including intuitive skills, to the full, at the same time applying her scientific knowledge in every situation.

REFERENCES

Bennett V R, Brown L K (eds) 1993 Myles textbook for midwives, 12th edn. Churchill Livingstone, Edinburgh

Bevis R 1984 Anaesthesia in midwifery. Bailliere Tindall, London

Brazelton T B 1973 Neonatal behavioural assessment scale. Clinics in developmental medicine 50. Heinemann, London

Browne D, Powell H 1993 Update on some earlier controversies. In: Morgan B M (ed) Controversies in obstetric anaesthesia No 2. Edward Arnold, London

Chamberlain G, Wraight A, Steer P (eds) 1993 Pain and its relief in childbirth. Churchill Livingstone, Edinburgh

Collins M K, Porter K B, Brook E et al 1994 Vulvar application of lidocaine for pain relief in spontaneous vertex delivery. Obstetrics and Gynecology 84 (3): 335–337

Davies G K, Tolhurst-Cleaver C L, James T L 1980 Respiratory depression after intrathecal narcotics. Anaesthesia 35: 1080–1083

Gordon S C, Gaines S K, Pickett Hauber R 1994 Self-administered versus nurse-administered epidural analgesia after Caesarian section. Journal of Obstetric, Gynecological and Neonatal Nursing 23 (2): 99–103

Haire D 1993 Update on obstetric related drugs and procedures: weighing the benefits against the risks. Proceedings of the International Confederation of Midwives, Vancouver 2: 793–797

Herz A (ed) 1993 Opioids (2 vols), Handbook of experimental pharmacology. Springer-Verlag, Berlin

Jacobsen B, Nyberg K, Gronbladh L et al 1990 Opiate addiction in adult offspring through possible imprinting after obstetric treatment. British Medical Journal 301 (6760): 1067–1070

Kuhnert B R, Linn P, Kennard M J et al 1985 Effects of low doses of meperidine on neonatal behaviour. Anesthesia and Analgesia 64: 335–342

Leicht C H, Hughes S C, Dailey P A et al 1986 Epidural morphine sulfate for analgesia after Caesarian section. Anaesthesiology 65: 366

McIntosh D G, Rayburn W F 1991 Patient controlled analgesia in obstetrics and gynecology. Obstetrics and Gynecology 78 (6): 1129–1135

MacLeod K 1993 Epidural opiates should be abandoned in obstetric patients – the arguments against. In: Morgan B M (ed) Controversies in obstetric anaesthesia, no 2. Edward Arnold, London

Morgan B M 1982 Double blind comparison of meptazinol and pethidine for relief of pain in labour. British Journal of Obstetrics and Gynaecology 89: 318–322

Morgan B M 1990 Changes in attitude towards pain relief in labour. Journal of Obstetrics and Gynaecology 10 (3): 236–237

Morgan B M, Bulpitt C J, Clifton P et al 1982 Analgesia and satisfaction in childbirth (the Queen Charlottes 1000 mother survey). Lancet ii: 808–810

Morrison J C et al 1973 Metabolites of meperidine related to fetal depression. American Journal of Obstetrics and Gynecology 15: 1132–1137

Osler M 1987 A double blind study comparing meptazinol and pethidine for relief of pain in labour. European Journal of Obstetrics and Gynaecology 26: 15–18

Priest J, Rosser J 1991 Pethidine–A shot in the dark (editorial) MIDIRS Midwifery Digest 1 (4): 373–375

Rajan L 1994 The impact of obstetric procedures and analgesia and anaesthesia during labour and delivery on breast feeding. Midwifery 10: 87–103

Rang H P, Dale M M, Ritter J M 1995 Pharmacology, 3rd edn. Churchill Livingstone, Edinburgh

Ranta P, Jouppila P, Spalding M et al 1995 Paracervical block – a viable alternative for labor pain relief? Acta Obstetrica and Gynecologica Scandinavica 72 (2): 122–126

Rayburn W, Leuschen M P, Earl R et al 1989 Intravenous meperidine during labor: a randomised comparison between nursing and patient controlled administration. Obstetrics and Gynecology 74 (5): 702–706

Report on the confidential enquiry into maternal deaths 1985–1987. HMSO, London

Reynolds F 1990a It is essential that antacid prophylaxis is given to all women in labour–arguments against. In: Morgan B M (ed) Controversies in obstetric anaesthesia, no 1. Edward Arnold, London

Reynolds F 1990b Pain relief in labour. British Journal of Obstetrics and Gynaecology 97: 757–759

Reynolds F 1993 Pain relief in labour. British Journal of Obstetrics and Gynaecology 100: 979–983

Rickford W J K, Reynolds F 1987 Expectations and experiences of pain relief in labour. In: Society for Obstetric Anaesthesia and Perinatology (Abstracts), Halifax, Nova Scotia, 163

Sheikh A, Tunstall M E 1986 Comparative study of meptazinol and pethidine for the relief of pain in labour. British Journal of Obstetrics and Gynaecology 93: 264–269

Steer P 1993 The methods of pain relief used. In: Chamberlain G, Wraight A, Steer P (eds) Pain and its relief in childbirth. Churchill Livingstone, Edinburgh

Thomson A M, Hillier V F 1994 A re-evaluation of the effect of pethidine on the length of labour. Journal of Advanced Nursing 19 (3): 448–456

Vella L, Francis D, Houlton P, Reynolds F 1985 Comparison of anti-emetics metoclopramide and promethazine in labour. British Medical Journal 290: 1173–1175

Wagner M 1993 Research shows medication of pain is not 'safe'. Caduceus 20: 14–15

Wee M Y K, Hasan M A, Thomas T A Isoflurane in labour. Anaesthesia 48 (5): 369–372

Woods S 1993 Epidural opiates should be abandoned in obstetric patients – arguments for. In: Morgan B M (ed) Controversies in obstetric anaesthesia, no 2. Edward Arnold, London

UKCC 1992 Standards for the administration of medicines. UKCC, London

UKCC 1993 Midwives' rules. UKCC, London

UKCC 1994 The midwife's code of practice. UKCC, London

FURTHER READING

Bennett V R, Brown L K 1993 The midwife. In: Bennett V R, Brown L K (eds) Myles textbook for midwives, 12th edn. Churchill Livingstone, Edinburgh

Bent E A 1993 Statutory control of the practice of midwives. In: Bennett V R, Brown L K (eds) Myles textbook for midwives 12th edn. Churchill Livingstone, Edinburgh

Bevis R 1984 Anaesthesia in midwifery. Bailliere Tindall, London

Dickersin K 1989 Pharmacological control of pain during labour. In: Chalmers I, Enkin M, Kierse M J N C (eds) Effective care in pregnancy and childbirth. Oxford University Press, Oxford

Heywood A M, Ho E 1990 Pain relief in labour. In: Alexander J, Levy V, Roch S (eds) Midwifery practice – intrapartum care. MacMillan Press, London

Laurence D R, Bennett P N 1987 Clinical pharmacology 6th edn. Churchill Livingstone, Edinburgh

Ostheimer G W (ed) 1992 Manual of obstetric anesthesia, 2nd edn. Churchill Livingstone, New York

Niven C 1990 Coping with labour pain – the midwife's role. In: Robinson S, Thomson A M (eds) Midwives, research and childbirth 3. Chapman and Hall, London

Roch S 1993 The use of drugs by the midwife. In: Bennett V R, Brown L K (eds) Myles textbook for midwives, 12th edn. Churchill Livingstone, Edinburgh

12

Regional anaesthesia: epidural and spinal block

Ruth Bevis

LEARNING OUTCOMES

At the end of this chapter the reader will have

- **an awareness of the views of women who may choose regional anaesthesia for labour**

- **a knowledge of the role and responsibilities of the midwife in relation to the administration of regional anaesthetics**

- **an increased awareness of the role of the anaesthetist and the procedure for epidural block**

- **an understanding of different types of regional anaesthesia including epidural block and 'mobile epidurals', spinal anaesthesia, caudal block**

- **considered some of the major research evidence and reports relating to the use of anaesthetics in labour.**

INTRODUCTION

When epidural anaesthesia was introduced in obstetric practice it was hailed as the ultimate pain relief for childbirth. Its widespread use began in the early 1970s as childbirth became a more medically managed event, with the emphasis on hospital as the only safe place for delivery. In 1970, the Central Midwives Board for England and Wales (CMB) passed a ruling allowing midwives to 'top-up' epidurals after suitable training and supervision. This was an important factor in the growth of epidural services.

In the early days of its use the epidural was a relatively simple matter of placing an epidural catheter in the epidural space. The drug used was a local anaesthetic agent, most commonly bupivacaine, in one of two or three concentrations. This had its limitations and disadvantages, and the technique continues to be refined and developed in order to meet the full range of women's needs. An important development in the 1990s is the 'mobile epidural', enabling women to have adequate analgesia with little or no motor block so that they may move around during their labour. At the other end of the spectrum is the epidural block for Caesarean section, where good anaesthesia is required for the challenge of abdominal surgery, with handling of uterus and intestines, and possible spillage of liquor and blood into the peritoneal cavity, all of which cause acute pain.

Anaesthesia and analgesia

It is important to differentiate between the terms anaesthesia and analgesia. Analgesia means relief of pain, but not necessarily loss of sensation. Anaesthesia means loss of sensation, including the sensation of pain. In local anaesthesia, loss of sensation is achieved in a small area, for example in infiltration of the perineum. In regional anaesthesia, loss of sensation is achieved in a larger area of the body, for example in epidural or spinal anaesthesia.

In general anaesthesia the subject is unconscious, and it is the responsibility of the anaesthetist to ensure that he or she is pain-free, since this is not necessarily the case. This is a particular hazard in general anaesthesia for Caesarean section, as the anaesthetist aims to avoid sedation and respiratory depression in the neonate.

Women and their views

Women approach labour and the relief of labour pain with a diversity of views. There is a tendency to believe that all sane women must want complete abolition of labour pain, but this is not the case. Some women do indeed want complete abolition of pain from the earliest possible stage, but others want the satisfaction of labouring without any kind of pharmacological help. They want to be sure that there will be no adverse effects on the baby or themselves, and they want to be fully alert and in control. Control is an important factor in a satisfying experience of childbirth, and in the days of routine enemas, perineal shaving and banning of partners from the labour room, control was completely removed from the woman.

The more passive woman may not be confident to make her own decisions and wants the locus of control to be maintained by others. She is happy to be 'managed' and will often accept advice unquestioningly (Kitzinger 1987, Poore & Cameron Foster 1989). The 'Facilitator' type (Raphael-Leff 1991) wants to make her own decisions and have the locus of control centred within herself; she will be disappointed, even devastated, if she does not achieve this (see Ch. 4).

With women having the choice of controlling their fertility, and generally having babies when they plan to do so, much more tends to be invested in each baby, and each labour is required to be a good and meaningful experience. Delivery has become a major life event with intense personal significance (Kitzinger 1987), which contrasts significantly with the acceptance by an earlier generation that repeated pregnancies, wanted or not, were an inevitable part of the 'woman's lot'.

Anecdotal evidence (Naulty 1990a) suggests that when one group of women receive a continuous epidural infusion, and a similar group receive a similar infusion at a slower rate with a patient-controlled analgesia (PCA) top-up facility, including a sub-group whose PCA button was programmed not to deliver any solution, the PCA group reported better analgesia than the group who did not have a PCA facility. The conclusion is that if women are given control they tend to report greater satisfaction even if labour does not progress as they had planned or hoped.

A woman may approach labour with an unrealistic view of the level, intensity and duration of the pain involved. It may be that her anticipation of the pain is realistic, but she over-estimates her ability to cope with it (Rickford & Reynolds 1987). Women who plan to use active coping techniques such as relaxation, TENS and full mobility during labour, and who then find themselves driven by pain and distress to accept an epidural, may feel an enduring sense of failure and dissatisfaction. A sensitive midwife will aim to minimise this, and can encourage the woman to resume control as far as possible once she is free of pain, particularly if the labour can then proceed without further medical intervention. The woman may need time after the labour for 'debriefing', and to discuss the details of her labour. When women are kept fully informed and come to joint decisions with the professionals, their distress and disappointment is likely to be minimised.

In evaluating the success of an epidural block it is the mother's report of satisfaction which is the goal, even if the block does not achieve clinically complete analgesia.

The midwife's role

The midwife has an important role as educator and advocate in enabling women to have access to the type of pain relief they require. If a woman is exhausted by several hours of labour and wishes respite and sleep in order to cope with the final stages, she needs good analgesia, but not necessarily a lot of fine tuning with regard to concentration, dosage or body position, in order for her to be up and about at that point in time. The midwife may need to encourage the anaesthetist to be sensitive to that woman's needs. She will also need to support and encourage the woman who had been determined not to have an epidural but who finds that her planned course of action is not appropriate. The midwife is a key person in the woman's birth experience, and her attitude and actions will be long remembered, even though other events are not.

Although the ultimate responsibility for the management of the epidural lies with the anaesthetist, it is the midwife who is alongside the woman, and she must continually be aware of the woman's analgesic needs. She must be able to recognise inadequacies in the analgesia which the anaesthetist may be able to remedy, such as a missed segment block (where analgesia is good on one side of the abdomen, but pain is felt on the

other). If pain is felt despite a continuous epidural infusion, a bolus top-up may be required.

THE EPIDURAL BLOCK
Procedure

The anaesthetist should talk to the woman requesting epidural analgesia and obtain her informed consent, explaining the procedure and pointing out its advantages and disadvantages. Informed consent, whatever the procedure, is an issue which has been widely discussed in many areas. Midwives should be aware of the legal issues and debates (Gild 1989). The midwife and anaesthetist should aim to judge each situation together with the woman and her partner, and give as much information as they require before proceeding.

Before initiating epidural analgesia the anaesthetist inserts an intravenous cannula. It is usual to give a 'preload' of intravenous fluid, such as 500 ml of Hartmann's solution. This is given because the local anaesthetic agents such as bupivacaine cause sympathetic as well as sensory and motor block, and this may cause hypotension which if untreated could lead to reduced placental perfusion and fetal hypoxia. Some anaesthetists question the need for this now, and it may not always be standard practice if local anaesthetic agents are combined with opioids or are used in very dilute solutions (Scott 1993). It is important that the intravenous cannula is in place so that intravenous fluid may be given if necessary. Ephedrine should always be readily available in case an acute drop in blood pressure does occur, especially when the epidural is being given prior to Caesarean section.

The anaesthetist may want the woman to sit upright with her back to him and her buttocks on the edge of the bed, or to lie in the left lateral position with her back curved as much as possible. This is very difficult for the woman in labour, if she is having strong, frequent contractions, and she will require much support and encouragement.

The anaesthetist scrubs and puts on a sterile gow 1 and gloves. The woman's back is sprayed with a skin cleaning agent, such as chlorhexidine in spirit. The back is then covered with sterile surgical towels.

The anaesthetist then infiltrates the skin and underlying tissues with local anaesthetic. (The underlying tissues are a small fat layer, supraspinous and intraspinous ligaments, and the ligamentum flavum which is thick and strong). A small 'nick' in the skin over lumbar vertebrae L 1–2, L 2–3, L 3–4 or occasionally L 4–5, enables the anaesthetist to insert the Tuohy needle. (Fig. 12.1 shows sites at which pain may be intercepted by local anaesthetic for various procedures, including epidural block.)

Throughout the procedure the anaesthetist will ask the woman herself—or the midwife if the woman is not able to respond—to inform him when a contraction is starting, and will then wait until it recedes. This is technically because the woman may move suddenly, increasing the risk of puncturing the dura mater, and because the epidural veins become distended during uterine contractions and the risk of puncturing one is greater, but it is also kinder to the labouring woman.

The anaesthetist then advances the Tuohy needle, attached to a free moving syringe, slowly and carefully. He depresses the syringe plunger gently to feel for the sensation of resistance as the needle tip reaches the ligamentum flavum, followed by loss of resistance as it enters the epidural space (a special plastic device to test for 'loss of resistance' is used; glass syringes are now rarely used for this part of the procedure). This is

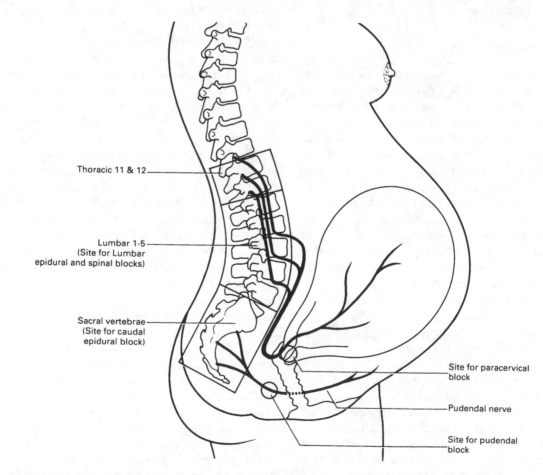

Figure 12.1 Pain pathways in labour, showing the sites at which pain may be intercepted by local anaesthetic technique (reproduced with kind permission from Bevis 1984).

the stage at which the dura mater may be punctured inadvertently, causing leakage of cerebrospinal fluid (CSF), and the anaesthetist will check that no drops of CSF appear at the end of the Tuohy needle. This accident is known as a dural tap. It is also possible to puncture an epidural vein, causing a 'bloody tap'. If either event occurs the epidural is resited.

The Tuohy needle is designed to direct the epidural catheter 'cephalad' (towards the woman's head) or 'caudad' (towards the base of her spine). The anaesthetist injects a test dose of anaesthetic solution, threads the epidural catheter through the Tuohy needle, holds it carefully in place, and withdraws the Tuohy needle once he is satisfied that the solution is in the epidural space.

The catheter is then strapped firmly in place, an antibacterial filter is attached to its distal end, and it is connected to a syringe driver if a continuous epidural infusion is to be used.

The anaesthetist's responsibility

The anaesthetist is responsible for observing the effects of the test dose. A sudden drop in blood pressure, together with rapid onset of extensive anaesthesia, indicates an undetected dural tap and 'inadvertent spinal'. An epidural dose of local anaesthetic such as 0.5% bupivacaine given into the CSF is potentially fatal, although a dilute solution is not so dangerous. In current anaesthetic practice, inadvertent spinal tap should never be fatal if it is managed correctly. Any complaints of generalised tingling or numbness, or of tinnitus may indicate intravenous injection of local anaesthetic.

The anaesthetist is responsible for prescribing top-ups, specifying the drug dosage and concentration, the frequency of top-ups, and the position the woman is to assume during the top-up. If a solution involving mixing of drugs and dilution is prescribed, the anaesthetist will be required to draw this up. The syringe must be clearly labelled with the woman's name, date and time of mixing, and contents. It must be kept beside the woman for whom it is prescribed, and carefully checked when administered.

Anaesthetists must be readily available, with the delivery suite as their top priority, whenever epidural anaesthesia is administered. They must attend if the midwife reports any inadequacy of the epidural, or if any complications arise.

The midwife's responsibility

The midwife has a clearly stated responsibility to ensure that she has been properly trained and supervised before she cares for a woman with an epidural. She must have a clear understanding of the procedure, be able to recognise any complications and take prompt, appropriate action.

If she is required to top up epidurals she must ensure that she is properly trained in this procedure and that she maintains her professional competence. As with the administration of any drugs, she must be familiar with the mode of action, the route of delivery, dosages, side-effects and signs of toxicity or overdosage.

She must monitor the condition of both mother and fetus, and the progress of the labour, and must follow any prescribed protocols or guidelines laid down in her place of work.

Care of the woman

The midwife must record the blood pressure at regular intervals, as prescribed in local protocol, or more frequently if prescribed or indicated. She should encourage the woman to empty her bladder every 2 hours, and keep a record of fluid intake and output. She should help the woman to maintain a comfortably supported position, ensuring that no damage occurs to the back or to numb legs. She should monitor the fetal heart as appropriate.

Mode of action

The epidural space is described as a potential space. The dural sac is closely apposed to the walls of the vertebral canal, and the space is only created by the injection of fluid or air into the epidural area (Bromage 1978). It contains fat and blood vessels; the spinal nerves enter and leave the spinal cord laterally through the epidural space. Local anaesthetic and opioid agents attach to receptor cells on the spinal nerves so that a particular area may be targeted for anaesthesia. The potential of the epidural space is slightly smaller in later pregnancy, due to venous congestion. The congestion increases as uterine contractions occur (see also Gaynor 1990).

Drugs used

Local anaesthetic agents

The anaesthetic agent most commonly used in the UK for epidural block is bupivacaine (Marcain). Lignocaine (Xylocaine or Lidocaine) may also be used; it gives analgesia very quickly, but its effect is relatively short-lived, so that there is a danger of cumulative effect and toxicity. Lignocaine is sometimes mixed with adrenaline and bicarbonate to provide a more rapid and dense block, particularly for Caesarean section.

Bupivacaine in a dextrose solution has a higher specific gravity than the CSF and therefore sinks to the lowest point in the subarachnoid space. Positioning of the subject is then crucial to the site of the block. Such spinal solutions are known as hyperbaric or 'heavy' solutions and are used *only* for spinal blocks, whereas plain bupivacaine is used for epidural blocks. Plain bupivacaine is sometimes used by a few anaesthetists for spinal blocks, although it is generally believed that this is rather dangerous because of the risk of a high block and respiratory embarrassment.

In some countries such as the USA, other local anaesthetic agents may be used in the subarachnoid space for spinal blocks (see p. 172). These may include cinchocaine (Nupercaine) and amethocaine (Tetracaine, Pontocaine) although these are not available in the UK for spinal blocks. These drugs are also available in a hyperbaric solution. Isobaric solutions, with a similar specific gravity to CSF spread more generally in the CSF and tend to give a wider area of less effective anaesthesia. Again there is a risk of high spread causing respiratory embarrassment.

Local anaesthetic agents work by blocking nervous impulses along nerve fibres. At rest the nerve cell is positively charged. When a nerve impulse travels along the fibre there is a rapid rise in the permeability of the cell membrane to sodium, caused by the 'sodium pump', and sodium enters the cell. Sodium is positively charged, and displaces the negatively charged potassium within the cell. This process is called depolarisation; it occurs along the entire nerve fibre, and at the neuromuscular junction it activates a neurotransmitter, acetylcholine. Local anaesthetic agents block the action of the sodium pump and therefore block the transmission of nerve impulses.

Opioid drugs (see also Ch. 11)

A variety of opioid drugs have been used in the epidural space, and although they produce good analgesia generally, they are not effective in labour. A combination of opioid and local anaesthetic is very effective. An opioid often used in the epidural space is fentanyl (Sublimaze). This is a synthetic opiate with good analgesic properties, but it is a potent respiratory depressant. Other opioids used include sufentanil, alfentanil, morphine, diamorphine and pethidine. Any epidural opioid is used with caution if the woman has already received pethidine or a similar drug during labour.

The main side-effects are nausea, sleepiness and generalised itching, which may be very troublesome. Bladder function may also be affected, leading to urinary retention. Naloxone is effective as an opioid antagonist when opioids are given by the epidural route, but as in any other situation, the undesirable side-effects are alleviated and the analgesic effect diminished.

Some anaesthetists are concerned that a degree of respiratory depression may occur, in some cases hours after epidural administration of opioids, and they feel that observing the woman's respiratory rate hourly is an inadequate method of detection (Woods 1993). It is thought that opioids may diffuse into the epidural veins, and they are known to diffuse into the CSF. There is concern that vomiting (which may be a side-effect of the opioid drug), coughing and pushing in the second stage may cause upward spread within the CSF and thus respiratory depression (Woods 1993). Others (MacLeod 1993) feel that the benefits far outweigh the disadvantages, and that the risks are minimal. The midwife must be aware of these risks, particularly when opioids are given for analgesia after Caesarean section, and must be vigilant in her observation of the woman. It is perhaps on the busy postnatal ward that respiratory depression is most likely to be missed.

Local anaesthetic and opioid combinations

It has been clearly shown that local anaesthetic and opioid agents used alone each has drawbacks and inadequacies, but a combination of the two has been shown to be very effective. Vella et al (1988) showed that combining the two drugs in the regional block was more effective than using a local anaesthetic drug in the epidural space preceded by a systemic opioid (intravenous fentanyl).

The two types of drug potentiate each other. The local anaesthetic tends to block the A delta fibres more effectively, while the opioid acts mainly on the C fibres. The resulting block gives better analgesia, although the local anaesthetic is used in a more dilute solution. Motor block is reduced, giving better mobility and greater sensation, and therefore more effective pushing in the second stage. Sympathetic block is reduced so that hypotension is less of a problem. (Murphy et al 1991, Naulty 1990b).

Indications for epidural block

Maternal request. This is the most common indication for an epidural.

Complications of labour. In cases such as malpresentation, malposition, premature labour or multiple pregnancy, all of which may necessitate instrumental delivery or Caesarean section, it may be advisable to have an epidural block. In addition, epidural block may be indicated for intrauterine death, minimising the emotional trauma which may be increased by the physical pain experienced in labour.

Pregnancy-induced hypertension. In this instance, the aim is to reduce stress from pain—with the resultant rise in circulating catecholamines—and to give effective analgesia for instrumental or operative delivery if this is neces-

sary. The epidural is not given to reduce the blood pressure, but to help prevent it rising further.

Medical conditions such as diabetes and cardiovascular, renal and respiratory disorders. Again the aim is to reduce stress and to give good analgesia for a possible assisted delivery. Epidural analgesia is generally advantageous for such women, although every case must be assessed carefully by the medical and anaesthetic teams. It is believed that most women with a medical condition will benefit from epidural analgesia (Macdonald 1990).

Contraindications

Contraindications are usually categorised as absolute or relative.

Absolute contraindications

There are some women who are not able to have an epidural, but the main absolute contraindication is maternal refusal.

Blood loss for any reason is another absolute contraindication because of the hypotension which follows epidural anaesthesia. Any woman with a coagulation problem is usually considered unsuitable for an epidural because of the risk of an epidural haematoma, which may cause pressure on the spinal cord resulting in paralysis.

An epidural is also contraindicated if there is any form of local sepsis or generalised infection, because of the risk of spread of infection in the form of an epidural abscess or meningitis.

Inadequate staffing levels or inadequate facilities are also an absolute contraindication.

Relative contraindications

Neurological problems such as multiple sclerosis have been cited as absolute contraindications to epidural analgesia in the past, because of the fear of any subsequent worsening of the condition being attributed to the epidural. It is now generally considered that as long as the woman is counselled well during pregnancy, understands the risks and benefits and makes an informed choice, good analgesia is of overall benefit. Any chronic back disorder or previous back surgery would be regarded similarly, and each case is considered individually (Macdonald 1990).

Advantages

The clear advantage of an epidural which is appropriately administered and effective is good pain relief. With an epidural catheter in place the epidural may be topped up for instrumental or operative delivery, or a more dilute dose of anaesthetic solution may be given for the second stage of labour.

Disadvantages

The main disadvantage voiced by women is their lack of mobility.

Epidural anaesthesia has been said to lead to a 'cascade of intervention', and certainly the use of the epidural inevitably involves the use of further technology. Until recently the woman with an epidural was confined to bed, had continuous fetal monitoring, a continuous intravenous infusion, she was likely to experience some difficulty with micturition and was likely to be catheterised at least once. Women dislike the numbness of the legs, which makes them feel restricted and powerless. This effect is reduced with the use of more dilute solutions of local anaesthetic and with the addition of an opioid.

Too profound a block during the second stage abolishes any sense of the bearing-down reflex, and the epidural has been cited as the cause of a rise in incidence of instrumental delivery. This statistic improved when the second stage of labour was managed less aggressively and women were not urged to push immediately full dilatation was recognised. Defining passive and active phases of the second stage has lengthened the second stage but does not appear to have an adverse effect on the fetus, and some studies report a reduction in the need for neonatal resuscitation. (Buxton & Redman 1990, Walkinshaw & Crosfill 1990).

It is generally unacceptable to give total pain relief during the first stage of labour and then allow the epidural to wear off for the second stage if full pain sensation then returns before delivery. If the epidural is managed in this way it is very difficult to predict subsequent events accurately. It is generally unnecessary with local anaesthetic and opioid combinations. (Carli 1990).

The epidural block may be patchy, so that good analgesia is not achieved over the entire lower abdomen and back. Good analgesia may be achieved on one side only—a missed segment block. This is very distressing, and women often say they would have preferred not to have an epidural at all. The reasons for these phenomena are not clear, but they may be due to some anomaly in the epidural space.

Puerperal and long-term sequelae

Unwelcome side-effects may occur during the puerperium; these may include urinary retention, backache or pain, perineal pain and dizziness. Repeated catheterisation may lead to urinary tract infection, with its associated long-term effects in some cases. Backache appears to be a long-term sequel for some women, and may be related to difficulty in inserting the epidural, or to more than one attempt being made (MacArthur et al 1990, Clark & McQueen 1993, Russell et al 1993). Maternal morbidity in the first year after childbirth is poorly understood, under-researched, and is probably more extensive than is appreciated at present.

Psychological effects may be attributed to the use of epidurals according to some writers. Some women may regard the epidural as removing control from them, while others may recognise that relief of their pain and distress reinstated at least a degree of control and dignity to them.

Complications

Early complications may include:

* Hypotension.
* Inadvertent intravascular or intrathecal injection.
* A dural tap occurs when the dura mater is punctured inadvertently during the insertion of

the epidural. Leakage of CSF occurs, and this may cause a 'spinal headache'. This distressing symptom is relieved by lying flat, but this makes early care of the baby very difficult. As soon as the woman sits up the headache returns in full intensity. It may be prevented or minimised at the time of the incident by infusing intravenous fluid into the epidural space, usually following delivery. If the headache is very severe or persists into the fourth or fifth day of the puerperium, a 'blood patch' may be performed. Venous blood is taken from the woman under strict asepsis by the anaesthetist, and injected into the epidural space via a Tuohy needle. The clotting of the blood is thought to seal the hole in the dura mater and to stop further leakage of CSF, and it often cures the headache within a very short time. The woman lies flat for about half an hour so that this can occur. When a dural tap occurs the epidural may be re-sited at another intervertebral space. A bloody tap occurs if an epidural vein is punctured during insertion of the epidural. It is recognised when blood is drawn back in the Tuohy needle. The epidural is then re-sited, usually without any adverse effects. Other later complications which every midwife needs to be aware of may include epidural haematoma or epidural abscess; careful observation of an uncomfortable or painful epidural site is therefore essential.

'MOBILE' EPIDURALS

Mobile epidural techniques have been devised to reduce the problems of heavy, immobile legs, and the lack of freedom to move, both of which were problems voiced by women. This can be a combined epidural/spinal technique (Morgan 1993b). The combination of local anaesthetic and opioid drugs gives good analgesia with less motor and sympathetic block. Each drug potentiates the other, so that lower doses of both are needed, in turn reducing side-effects. When any sensation begins to return a top-up should be given, since the analgesia is necessarily light and wears off quickly. If the local anaesthetic and opioid drugs are given in a large volume of normal saline, so that the solution is very dilute, there is a risk of cumulative effect over time if top-ups are given

too frequently. However, the drugs in this dilution are reported to be very safe even if accidentally given intrathecally or intravenously. The mobile epidural does not give full, unlimited mobility and the woman must be acquainted with this beforehand. The woman must be carefully monitored and observed since there will be some reduction in motor function and hypotension could still occur. To assess the woman's motor function, the midwife presses on the woman's thighs, and asks her to raise her legs from the bed. Telemetry may be used to monitor the fetal heart as necessary.

METHODS OF ADMINISTRATION OF EPIDURAL ANAESTHESIA

There are three main methods of administering epidural anaesthesia. These are continuous epidural infusion, patient-controlled epidural analgesia (PCEA) and intermittent bolus top-ups. All of these methods require an epidural catheter. It is possible, but not common in obstetrics, to give a 'single shot' epidural for a short period of effective analgesia; in this case the anaesthetic solution is given through the Tuohy needle and no epidural catheter is inserted.

Continuous infusion gives a steady background analgesia and may be augmented by a bolus top-up given by the anaesthetist as required, or by a series of regular, timed top-ups (Purdy et al 1987). PCEA is very satisfactory for many women (Fontenot et al 1993). There are the built-in safeguards of a controlled dose which may only be repeated after a certain period of time. If this dose proves inadequate, the anaesthetist may give a bolus top-up which often boosts the analgesia effectively. It is very important that the infusion equipment used for both methods is checked and maintained at regular intervals, and the midwife must observe the infusion rate during labour, to check that the equipment is functioning correctly. Toxicity and overdosage have not been shown to be a problem except when infusions are continued for more than 12 hours. (Li et al 1985, Gaylard et al 1987). Fairly extensive training is required for midwives in order to manage PCEA safely. Another factor, which many cost-conscious managers will be aware of, is that the machines are extremely expensive to purchase. Intermittent bolus top-ups do not give a continuous level of analgesia, and the effect has been described as 'roller coaster analgesia' (Gaylard 1990).

The midwife and top-ups

The midwife's responsibilities and professional accountability in caring for women with epidurals have already been discussed (see p. 167).

The topping up of an epidural is a procedure which must not be approached lightly. The top-up should be given promptly to prevent an overwhelming return of pain sensation. Ideally it should be given as soon as any significant return of sensation is reported.

The midwife checks that the epidural catheter has not become displaced and that there is no blood in the lumen. She then checks that the intravenous infusion is running freely. She checks the prescription and dose with another midwife, and draws it up if appropriate, or checks the amount to be given if a mixed solution has been prepared by the anaesthetist. She positions the woman as necessary. The position is usually prescribed by the anaesthetist. If it is not prescribed, the woman should not be lying on her side, but she must also not lie flat because of the risk of aortocaval occlusion and hypotension. A top-up for second stage, or to block the sacral nerves, is given with the woman sitting upright.

The fetal heart and maternal blood pressure are measured and recorded immediately afterwards, and at the prescribed intervals for the next 30 minutes. If there is any doubt at any stage of the procedure about any factor involved, the midwife must seek the advice of the anaesthetist and must record the fact in the notes. She must at all times be aware of any signs or symptoms of complications arising from the giving of drugs by the epidural route, and must have a clear understanding of these. Crawford (1985) stated that 'epidural analgesia for labour and delivery, including topping up by well-informed midwives, is characterised by an extremely high level of safety for the mother'.

CAUDAL BLOCK

This alternative epidural technique is not widely used in the UK for obstetrics, although it is more commonly used for children undergoing general surgery and for women for gynaecological surgery. It involves injecting local anaesthetic solution via the sacral hiatus, between the fifth sacral vertebra and the coccyx. The sacrococcygeal membrane overlies the sacral hiatus, and the epidural space lies beyond it. The dural sac, containing CSF, normally terminates at the level of the second sacral vertebra. It is possible to insert an epidural catheter via the caudal route, but the total dose of local anaesthetic dose required may be quite high, with the consequent risk of toxicity. The block produced tends to be lower, with abolition of the urge to bear down at full dilatation. Effective rapid sacral block for instrumental delivery is more commonly achieved by spinal anaesthesia.

SPINAL ANAESTHESIA

This is a different technique to epidural block. A much smaller dose of a different local anaesthetic agent is injected directly into the subarachnoid space, and therefore into the CSF.

Advantages

A rapid, effective block is achieved. The use of a small dose of local anaesthetic does not usually give rise to any side-effects, including significant hypotension, although the blood pressure must still be monitored carefully. The block may usually be determined very accurately by the use of hyperbaric anaesthetic solutions, and careful positioning of the woman.

Disadvantages

Puncturing the dura, with leakage of CSF, resulted in a spinal headache in a significant number of cases until the advent of very fine 'pencil point' spinal needles. The technique is normally a single shot procedure, with no facility for topping up, and therefore the effect is relatively short-lived.

This does not normally pose a problem for forceps or Ventouse delivery, or for manual removal of the placenta or suturing of a complicated perineal tear. Continuous spinal infusions are used, but this is not currently in wide use for labour. A combined epidural/spinal approach has been devised for Caesarean section (see below). There is total motor block of the anaesthetised area, but if a single shot is given, this is relatively short-lived, and this disadvantage is offset by the total anaesthesia which is achieved.

REGIONAL BLOCK FOR CAESAREAN SECTION

Lumbar epidural block is now widely used for Caesarean section. It allows the woman to be awake and alert, and to see and hold her baby very soon after delivery in most cases. In most centres in the UK the partner may also be present if the couple wish. It is safer than general anaesthesia. If an epidural for labour is in place and working well, it may usually be topped up quite quickly for Caesarean section. The use of a mixture of lignocaine and bupivacaine gives both rapid and sustained analgesia, and is favoured by some anaesthetists. Others will use a local anaesthetic and opioid mixture. The woman remains awake and alert in the postoperative period, with the facility for good postoperative analgesia via the epidural catheter. This facilitates early ambulation, with its associated reduction in complications following Caesarean section.

The block required is more extensive and more profound than for labour and vaginal delivery. The block must be fully effective from S5 to the level of T6. This means the woman will experience loss of sensation from the nipples down. If the block extends above this level there is the danger of respiratory difficulties. The block must be fully effective before surgery commences. The anaesthetist will test the level and effectiveness of the block by use of a cold spray, such as ethyl chloride, and by pin-prick. The feet and legs will become warm, indicating sympathetic blockade. This profound, extensive block is achieved by the use of larger doses of concentrated local anaesthetic agent, usually bupivacaine 0.5%. The sympathetic block may cause hypotension, and a preload of intravenous fluid is given before the epidural is commenced. Ephedrine must be available for immediate use intravenously if the blood pressure drops significantly. As stated previously, a mixture of lignocaine, adrenaline and bicarbonate is often used for epidural Caesarean section.

Spinal anaesthesia is now more commonly used for Caesarean section which is partly due to use of the 'pencil point' needles which produce a very low incidence of postdural headaches. A continuous infusion may be given through a very fine catheter. However, if a single shot technique is used its duration of action cannot be extended. A combined spinal/epidural technique has been developed. This means the woman can be given rapid anaesthesia by means of the spinal block, with the advantage of an epidural catheter for maintaining anaesthesia during surgery and giving effective postoperative analgesia. A Tuohy needle is introduced into the epidural space, and a fine spinal needle passed through it into the subarachnoid space. The subarachnoid dose is given and the spinal needle withdrawn. An epidural catheter is then inserted through the Tuohy needle before the Tuohy needle is removed.

Caesarean section under local anaesthesia

It is possible to perform Caesarean section under local anaesthesia. A number of sites must be infiltrated with local anaesthetic, including deeper tissues such as the rectus muscle. The effects on the fetus are reported to be minimal and the onset of anaesthesia is rapid, so that it may be useful in an emergency situation (Ostheimer 1992).

Regional blocks and the fetus and neonate

It is essential to consider the effect on the second half of the duo in obstetric anaesthesia/analgesia. Bupivacaine as used in current UK practice does not have any significant adverse effect on the fetus or neonate (Kuhnert et al 1984, Reynolds 1990). There may be changes in the cardiotocograph following administration of bupivacaine, however the incidence may be reduced by fluid preloading (Umstad et al 1993). Fetal well-being is assessed by means of cardiotocography, fetal blood sampling, or possibly by Doppler assessment of flow-velocity waveforms in the fetal arteries.

Neonatal behaviour and adaptation to extrauterine life is scrutinised using one of the current neurobehavioural assessment scales. These include the Brazelton neonatal behavioural assessment scale (BNBAS), the early neonatal neurobehavioural scale (ENNS), and the neurological and adaptive capacity score (NACS). All are designed to detect subtle drug effects. Overall, babies born by Caesarean section have better short-term scores after epidural than general anaesthetic (however, general anaesthetic is more likely to be used if there is severe fetal distress). After 24 hours there are no significant differences (Abboud et al 1985).

Breastfeeding has been found to be more quickly established, and for a longer period, in mothers who have an epidural for Caesarean section, compared with mothers who have a general anaesthetic (Lie & Juul 1988).

SAFETY AND EPIDURAL SERVICES

It is only safe to offer an epidural to every woman who requests it if the obstetric unit has a suitably experienced anaesthetist available, with the labour ward as the top priority throughout the 24-hour period. The anaesthetist must have the support of a senior anaesthetist available at all times, for advice and for immediate assistance when necessary. There must also be sufficient midwives, who are adequately trained and experienced, to care for the women receiving epidural anaesthesia.

THE SHORT (1980) REPORT

The Short committee sat during 1979–1980, looking at perinatal and neonatal mortality. A number of recommendations were made relating to obstetric anaesthetic services, recognising the link between skilled care for the mother and the outcome of delivery for the baby.

The recommendations were as follows:

• A 24-hour service for epidurals on request should be available as an important priority in consultant obstetric units.
• There should be immediate availability of anaesthetists to the delivery room.
• Every obstetric unit delivering more than 1000 women per year 'should have attached to it a consultant anaesthetist with at least two sessions of his contract committed to obstetric anaesthesia'. The number of sessions should be increased proportionately according to the number of deliveries per year.
• Midwives should be formally trained by anaesthetists to top up epidurals.

One of the conclusions of the report was that the provision of anaesthetic cover is still inadequate in some places, and epidurals 'on demand' are not available throughout the UK (Hibbard & Scott 1990, Chamberlain et al 1993).

THE OBSTETRIC ANAESTHETISTS' ASSOCIATION

Obstetric anaesthesia is now recognised as a speciality in its own right, and the Obstetric Anaesthetists' Association (OAA) meet, debate and publish material regularly. This provides a forum for stimulation, discussion and for sharing research and experiences (Morgan 1990, 1993b). There is room for debate, and opinions differ on many issues within the speciality, but members are committed to the safety and satisfaction of women in labour. There are specific hazards and potential problems relating to general anaesthesia for pregnant and newly delivered women, and anaesthetists are involved in high dependency care in the obstetric unit.

THE REPORT ON CONFIDENTIAL ENQUIRIES INTO MATERNAL DEATHS

This report is published every 3 years, and the past two have examined the available evidence from every maternal death in the UK; previous reports covered England and Wales. It is an important audit tool in obstetric care. The report makes sobering reading. The number of deaths attributed directly to general or regional anaesthesia has fallen over the years, from 27 in the report for 1973–1975, to four in the report for 1988–1990. Most maternal deaths are related to general anaesthesia, and so the increased use and refining of regional techniques have undoubtedly been a significant factor. In the report for 1988–1990, there were 10 deaths 'to which anaesthesia contributed', and a 'late death' (after 42 days post-delivery) was directly due to anaesthesia.

The report highlights substandard care in almost 50% of maternal deaths. The authors acknowledge and commend the increase in 'dedicated consultant sessions for obstetric anaesthetists' in the past 10 years, but still found evidence of inadequate supervision of junior staff. The report states that: 'Midwifery staff deputised to look after postoperative patients should be specifically trained in monitoring, the care of the airway and resuscitative procedures, and should be supervised by a defined anaesthetist at all times'.

Further centralisation of maternity services is advocated in order to provide adequate consultant cover. Midwives will wish to balance the need for safe services with the needs and wishes of the woman and her family. Much maternal morbidity and mortality is related to pre-existing disease or acute illness, and the main cause of death is severe haemorrhage. Recognition of risk factors during pregnancy is an important element in preventing the disasters outlined in the reports.

SUMMARY

Epidurals are doubtless becoming safer to use, as demonstrated by the trends in the report into maternal deaths. However, it is a complicated procedure which the midwife must become fully acquainted with if risks are to be minimised. Throughout the process of an epidural, the midwife must maintain professional competence and, to do this, she must be familiar with the mode of action, route of delivery and dosage, as well as the complications that might arise so that she can take prompt action if necessary.

It is also important for the midwife to be well acquainted with the various protocols and guidelines laid down at her place of work, so that she is aware of the framework within which she is operating. In this way, standards of safety will be maintained, if not improved.

REFERENCES

Abboud T K, Naggappala S, Murakawa K et al 1985 Comparison of effects of regional and general anaesthetic on neonatal neurologic and adaptive scores. Anesthesia and Analgesia 64: 996–1000
Bevis R 1984 Anaesthesia in midwifery. Balliere Tindall, London
Bromage P R 1978 Epidural analgesia. W B Saunders, Philadelphia
Buxton J, Redman C 1990 Effects of epidural analgesia and delayed pushing in the second stage on fetal condition. Contemporary Reviews in Obstetrics and Gynaecology 2 (2): 80–86
Carli F 1990 With-holding top-ups in the second stage is barbaric – arguments for. In: Morgan B M (ed) Controversies in obstetric anaesthesia, no 1. Churchill Livingstone, Edinburgh
Chamberlain G, Wraight A, Steer P 1993 Pain and its relief in childbirth. Churchill Livingstone, Edinburgh
Clark V A, McQueen M A 1993 Factors influencing backache following epidural analgesia in labour. International Journal of Obstetric Anesthesia 2 (4): 193–196
Crawford J S 1985 Some maternal complications of epidural analgesia for labour. Anaesthesia 40: 1219–1225
Fontenot R J et al 1993 Double-blind evaluation of patient-controlled epidural analgesia during labour. International Journal of Obstetric Anesthesia 2 (2): 73–77
Gaylard D G, Wilson I H, Balmer H G R 1987 An epidural infusion technique for labour. Anaesthesia 42: 1098–1101
Gaynor A 1990 The lumbar epidural region – anatomy and approach. In: Reynolds F (ed) Epidural and spinal blockade in obstetrics. Bailliere Tindall, London
Gild M W 1989 Informed consent – a review. Anesthesia and Analgesia 68: 649–653
Hibbard B M, Scott D B 1990 The availability of epidural anaesthesia and analgesia in obstetrics. British Journal of Obstetrics and Gynaecology 97 (5): 402–405
Kitzinger S 1987 Some women's experiences of epidurals: a descriptive study. National Childbirth Trust, London
Kuhnert B R, Harrison M J, Linn P L et al 1984 Effects of maternal epidural anaesthesia on neonatal behaviour. Anesthesia and Analgesia 63: 301–308
Li D F, Rees G A D, Rosen M 1985 Continuous extradural infusion of 0.0625% or 0.125% bupivacaine for pain relief in primigravid labour. British Journal of Anaesthesia 57: 264–270
Lie B, Juul J 1988 Effect of epidural versus general anaesthetic on breast feeding. Acta Obstetrica Gynaecologica Scandinavica 67: 207–209
MacArthur C, Lewis M, Knox E G et al 1990 Epidural anaesthesia and long-term back ache after childbirth. British Medical Journal 301: 9–12

Macdonald R 1990 Indications and contra-indications for epidural blockade in obstetrics. In: Reynolds F (ed) Epidural and spinal blockade in obstetrics. Bailliere Tindall, London

MacLeod K 1993 Epidural opiates should be abandoned in obstetric patients – arguments against. In: Morgan B M (ed) Controversies in obstetric anaesthesia, no 2. Edward Arnold, London

Morgan B M (ed) 1990 Controversies in obstetric anaesthesia, no 1. Edward Arnold, London

Morgan B M (ed) 1993b Controversies in obstetric anaesthesia, no 2. Edward Arnold, London

Morgan B M 1993a Mobile epidurals: combined spinal / epidural analgesia in labour. MIDIRS Midwifery Digest 3 (3): 312–313

Morgan B M, Bulpitt C J, Clifton P et al 1982 Analgesia and satisfaction in childbirth (the Queen Charlotte's 1000 mother survey). Lancet ii: 808–810

Morgan B M, Bulpitt C J, Clifton P et al 1984 The consumer's attitude to obstetric care. British Journal of Obstetrics and Gynaecology 90: 624–628

Murphy J D, Henderson K, Bowden M I et al 1991 Bupivacaine versus bupivacaine plus fentanyl for epidural analgesia: the effect on maternal satisafaction. British Medical Journal 302 (6776): 564–567

Naulty J S 1990a Discussion. In Morgan B M (ed) Controversies in obstetric anaesthesia, no 1. Edward Arnold, London

Naulty J S 1990b Epidural and spinal opiates in labour. In: Reynolds F (ed) Epidural and Spinal Blockade in Obstetrics. Bailliere Tindall, London

Ostheimer G W (ed) 1992 Manual of obstetric anesthesia 2nd edn. Churchill Livingstone, New York

Poore M, Cameron Foster J 1989 Epidural and no epidural anaesthesia: differences between mothers and their experience of birth. Birth 12: 205–213

Purdy G, Currie J, Owen H 1987 Continuous extradural analgesia in labour. British Journal of Anaesthesia 59: 319–324

Raphael-Leff J 1991 Psychological processes of childbearing. Chapman and Hall, London

Report on Confidential Enquiry into Maternal Deaths in the UK 1988–1990. HMSO, London

Reynolds F 1989 Epidural analgesia in obstetrics – pros and cons for mother and baby. British Medical Journal 299: 751–752

Reynolds F 1993 Pain relief in labour. British Journal of Obstetrics and Gynaecology 100: 979–983

Rickford W J K, Reynolds F 1987 Expectations and experiences of pain relief in labour. In: Society for Obstetric Anesthesia and Perinatology (abstracts). Halifax, Nova Scotia, p 163

Russell R, Groves P, Taub N et al 1993 Assessing longterm backache after childbirth. British Medical Journal 306 (6888): 1299–1303

Scott D 1993 Pre-loading prior to regional block is an old wives' tale – arguments for. In: Morgan B M (ed) Controversies in obstetric anaesthesia, no 2. Edward Arnold, London

Short R 1980 Second report from the social services committee on perinatal and neonatal mortality 1. HMSO, London

Umstad M P, Ross A, Rushford D D et al 1993 Epidural analgesia and fetal heart rate abnormalities. Australia and New Zealand Journal of Obstetrics and Gynaecology 33 (3): 269–272

Viscomi C, Eisenach J C 1991 Patient-controlled epidural analgesia during labour. Obstetrics and Gynecology 77 (3): 348–351

Walkinshaw S A, Crosfill F 1990 Labour with epidural analgesia: second thoughts about the second stage. Journal of Obstetrics and Gynaecology 10(6): 499–502

Woods S 1993 Epidural opiates should be abandoned in obstetric patients–arguments for. In: Morgan B M (ed) Controversies in Obstetric Anaesthesia No2. Edward Arnold, London

FURTHER READING

Carrie L E S 1987 Regional techniques in obstetrics. In: Wildsmith J A W, Armitage E N (eds) Principles and practice of regional anaesthesia. Churchill Livingstone, Edinburgh

Crawford J S 1982 Obstetric anaesthesia and analgesia. Current reviews in obstetrics and gynaecology, 1. Churchill Livingstone, Edinburgh

Doughty A 1987 Landmarks in the development of regional analgesia in obstetrics. In: Morgan B M (ed) Foundations of obstetric anaesthesia. Farrand Press, London

Mander R 1993 Epidural analgesia 1: recent history. British Journal of Midwifery 1 (6): 259–263

Mander R 1994 Epidural analgesia 2: research basis. British Journal of Midwifery 2 (1): 12–16

Meehan F P 1987 Historical review of caudal epidural analgesia in obstetrics. Midwifery 3 (1): 39–45

Moir D D, Thorburn J 1986 Obstetric anaesthesia and analgesia. Bailliere Tindall, London

Thorp J A, McNitt J D, Leppert P C 1990 Effects of epidural analgesia: some questions and answers. Birth 17 (3): 157–162

Index

Page numbers in bold type refer to illustrations and tables.